D1268892

THE
INJECTABLE
DRUG
REFERENCE

Mary Lea Gora-Harper, PharmD
Director, Drug Information Center
Associate Professor
Pharmacy Practice and Science
University of Kentucky
College of Pharmacy and Hospital
Lexington, Kentucky

Developed in conjunction with the
Society of Critical Care Medicine

Note: Every effort has been made to ensure the accuracy of medication dosages and treatment schedules in this book. Recommendations are in accordance with generally accepted usage at the time of publication. However, drug usage constantly changes as new information arises from research and clinical experience. Thus, the reader is advised to consult the package insert material for each drug. The author, publisher, editor, reviewers, and the Society of Critical Care Medicine cannot be held responsible for the continued currency of the information or for errors or omissions. They disclaim all responsibility for any liability, loss, injury, or damage incurred as a consequence, directly or indirectly, of the use and application of any of the contents of this volume.

1 2 3 4 5 6 7 8 9 10

ISBN 0-9655531-0-8

9 780965 553100   52995

THE INJECTABLE DRUG REFERENCE

REVIEWERS

This book was reviewed in conjunction with the following reviewers from the Society of Critical Care Medicine's Section of Clinical Pharmacology and Pharmacy.

CHAIR, REVIEW BOARD

Erkan Hassan, PharmD, FCCM
Associate Professor
University of Maryland School of Pharmacy
Adjunct Clinical Specialist in Critical Care
Department of Pharmacy Services
University of Maryland Medical Systems
Baltimore, Maryland

SECTION LEADERS

Mary Birmingham, PharmD
Assistant Professor
Program Director, Critical Care
State University of New York
    at Buffalo
Millard Fillmore Hospital
Buffalo, New York

Linda J. Pine, PharmD, BCPS
Critical Care Specialist
Division of Pharmaceutical
    Services
Emory University Hospital
Departments of Pharmacy,
    Anesthesia and Pulmonary
    Critical Care Medicine
Atlanta, Georgia

**Michael O'Neil, PharmD,
BCNSP**
Critical Care Specialist
Clinical Pharmacy Coordinator
Charleston Area Medical
    Center
Charleston, West Virginia

Maria Rudis, PharmD, BCPS
Assistant Professor
Clinical Pharmacy
    and Emergency Medicine
University of Southern
    California
Schools of Pharmacy and
    Medicine
Los Angeles, California

continued next page

SECTION PARTICIPANTS

Tracy Aber, PharmD, BCPS
Critical Care Specialist
Baylor University Medical
    Center
Dallas, Texas

Daniel H. Albrant, PharmD
President, Pharmacy Dynamics
Arlington, Virginia

Brian D. Buck, PharmD
Critical Care Specialist
University of Maryland Medical
    System
Baltimore, Maryland

Diann Clarens-Hoedl, PharmD
Medical Science Manager
Bristol-Myers Squibb
Milwaukee, Wisconsin

Brad E. Cooper, PharmD
Clinical Pharmacist
Division of Cardiology and
    Critical Care
Hamot Medical Center
Department of Pharmacy/Drug
    Information
Erie, Pennsylvania

Douglas N. Fish, PharmD
Assistant Professor
Clinical Specialist, Critical Care
Department of Pharmacy
    Practice
University of Colorado Health
    Sciences Center
School of Pharmacy
Denver, Colorado

Tracey L. Goldsmith, PharmD
Clinical Manager
Department of Pharmacy
Hermann Hospital
Houston, Texas

Mary Hess, PharmD
Critical Care Specialist
Department of Pharmacy
    Services
University of Pittsburgh
    Medical Center
Pittsburgh, Pennsylvania

Steven R. Kayser, PharmD
Clinical Professor
Department of Clinical
    Pharmacy
University of California
San Francisco, California

Christian Klem, PharmD
Critical Care Pharmacotherapy
    Specialist
Department of Pharmacotherapy
    and Research
Tampa General Health Care
Tampa, Florida

Vanessa L. Kluth, PharmD
Clinical Specialist, Critical Care
Department of Pharmacy
Hermann Hospital
Houston, Texas

**Kenneth R. Lawrence,
PharmD**
Manager, Clinical Pharmacy
    Services
SICU Pharmacist
Beth Israel Deaconess Medical
    Center
Boston, Massachusetts

Clyde I. Miyagawa, PharmD
Clinical Pharmacist Specialist
Division of Trauma/Critical Care
University Hospital
Department of Pharmacy
Cincinnati, Ohio

Lea Anne O'Brien, PharmD
Clinical Liaison
Roche Pharmaceuticals
Nutley, New Jersey

Ed Seidl, PharmD
Clinical Specialist, Critical Care
Department of Pharmacy
    Services
Allegheny General Hospital
Pittsburgh, Pennsylvania

**Catherine C. Turkel, PharmD,
FCCM**
Director of Drug Development
    and Data Management
Cypros Pharmaceutical
    Corporation
Carlsbad, California

CONTRIBUTING REVIEWER

Michael Collins, RPh
Distinguished Clinical Pharmacist
Clinical Assistant Professor of Pharmacy and Neurology
University of Wisconsin Hospital and Clinics
Madison, Wisconsin

TABLE OF CONTENTS

The drugs in this book are listed alphabetically by generic name. See the indexes in the back for listing by brand name and therapeutic category.

OVERVIEW

The Injectable Drug Reference is intended to be an easy-to-use, up-to-date, and practical pocket reference for reliable information on injectable medications frequently used in the critical care or emergency department. It can be used as a resource for nurses, pharmacists, physicians, or other health care professionals who are problem-solving with pharmacotherapeutic issues. It may be useful for the education of new practitioners or students practicing in acute care medicine.

This resource organizes and summarizes the crucial information on the indications, methods of administration, dosing and administration (including therapeutic drug monitoring information), monitoring parameters, and stability and compatibility information (pH, protect from light, solution compatibility, and drug compatibility). The information in *The Injectable Drug Reference* is organized into monographs covering approximately 100 commercially available medications sorted alphabetically by nonproprietary name.

If the medication is available only through one manufacturer in the United States, then the trade name and manufacturer are listed. If several manufacturers supply the product, then one common trade name and manufacturer will be listed, however, there will be an indication that various manufacturers supply the product. For those products with several manufacturers, the author does not endorse the use of any product over another, but rather is providing the reader who is less familiar with nonproprietary names with a common trade name. These trade names are also cross-referenced to nonproprietary names in the index. The monographs are divided into the following subheadings:

Methods of administration: describes frequently used injectable methods of administration (eg, direct intravenous injection and continuous infusion but not oral or rectal administration).

Dosing and administration: describes standard concentrations used for intravenous piggyback administration if applicable, and typical indications and doses for use in the intensive care unit or emergency department. Indications for another setting (eg, ambulatory chemotherapy) are not included.

Monitor: describes some parameters to monitor to assess safety and efficacy. If applicable, also describes therapeutic drug monitoring considerations (recommended times for blood sample collection and target serum levels).

Protect from light: describes whether medication needs to be protected from light. Information is based primarily on manufacturer recommendations.

Special considerations: describes issues in administration of medications including intravenous pump considerations or special information regarding administration.

pH: describes information provided on pH based primarily on manufacturer information.

Stability: describes information regarding general stability factors (eg, refrigeration requirements, color change indicator of instability).

Solution compatibility: lists compatibility information for several of the most common solutions. The following abbreviations are used in the text:

D_5W	Dextrose 5% in water
$D_{10}W$	Dextrose 10% in water
NS	Sodium chloride 0.9%
$D_5^{1}/_2NS$	Dextrose 5% in sodium chloride 0.45%
LR	Ringer injection, lactated

The absence of information implies neither compatibility nor incompatibility.

Compatible and incompatible (co-administration with other medications): a medication combination is considered compatible if information supports either physical or chemical compatibility with the other medication tested by y-site administration. A medication combination may be considered incompatible if scientific evidence supports either physical or chemical incompatibility tested in several conditions such as through y-site, syringe, or mixing the two medications.

The medication combinations that were researched from the literature are considered those primarily used in the acute care setting. The absence of compatibility information implies neither compatibility nor incompatibility of the combination. It may be that information is either lacking or controversial. This resource is a quick source for information and should not replace the use of textbooks such as *Handbook on Injectable Drugs* (American Society of Health-System Pharmacy) or *Injectable Drug Book*, nor examination of the primary literature to apply the information to a particular situation.

Many factors influence the compatibility of medications including drug concentration, pH, temperature, and order of mixing. And many of the trials examine only physical and not chemical compatibility, therefore, although the combination may not result in precipitation or haze, the literature may not address chemical decomposition. Readers are reminded that, if possible, medications should be administered separately to avoid risk of incompatibilities.

Accuracy of information: Every effort has been made to assure that the information contained within this publication is accurate and in accord with the standards accepted at the time of publication. However as new research and experience broaden our knowledge, changes in clinical practice, therapeutic intervention and drug interactions, and compatibility information occur. The reader is therefore advised to check, prior to the administration of any drug listed in this publication, the individual drug product information included in the packaging of each drug being considered for administration to be certain that changes have not been made that could modify the validity of the information contained herein.

ACETAZOLAMIDE
Diamox®, Lederle Laboratories, and other manufacturers

Methods of administration
Direct intravenous injection (100 mg/mL solution at 125 mg/minute), intermittent intravenous infusion (over 20 minutes), and intramuscular (causes pain on injection because of the alkaline pH)

Dosing and administration
Standard: 250 mg/50 mL of D_5W or NS (maximum concentration: 100 mg/mL)

Metabolic alkalosis or diuresis
Administer acetazolamide 250 mg every 8 to 12 hours to 500 mg every 12 to 24 hours by direct intravenous injection (maximum infusion rate 125 mg/minute) or by intermittent intravenous infusion. A maximum of 1 g/day should be used. Higher daily doses usually do not result in improved efficacy, but will increase the risk of side effects. Typically, patients are treated for up to 48 hours.

Acute closed-angle glaucoma
To facilitate rapid reduction in ocular tension (eg, preoperatively), administer 500 mg by direct intravenous injection, followed by 250 mg every 4 hours until desired effects are achieved. A dose of up to 1 g may be necessary to decrease intraocular pressure adequately.

General
Eliminate contributing factors of metabolic alkalosis, including correction of fluid status and electrolyte imbalance (eg, hypokalemia, hypochloremia, and hyponatremia); treat underlying cause. Acid losses can occur secondary to several causes, including vomiting, nasogastric suction, and diuretic use.

Patients with renal insufficiency may have variable diuretic response; adjust interval to every 12 hours in patients with a creatinine clearance less than 50 mL/minute. Avoid in patients with a creatinine clearance less than 10 mL/minute.

Monitor

Acid/base status (may take up to 12 hours to see significant correction of metabolic alkalosis; resolution of the signs of metabolic alkalosis include a decrease in blood pressure, cardiac arrhythmias, hypoventilation, and a decrease in ionized serum calcium), serum electrolytes (sodium, chloride, potassium [hypokalemia can occur with treatment]), complete blood cell count with differential, tachyphylaxis (typically seen after 48 hours of therapy; may require an acetazolamide-free period for up to 24 hours), allergic reactions (cross-reactivity with sulfonamides), fluid status (input and output), and serum creatinine.

May cause a metabolic acidosis with greatest risk in the elderly and in patients with renal impairment and diabetes mellitus. Signs and symptoms include myocardial depression, malaise, fatigue, myalgia, and hypotension.

May cause a decreased effect of some medications because of alkalization of urine (eg, quinidine, procainamide, and phenobarbital).

Protect from light: no

Special considerations: none

pH: 9.2 (after reconstitution with sterile water for injection)

Stability:

Less stable at pH >9; admixtures stable for up to 5 days at room temperature.

Solution compatibility: D_5W, NS, LR, D_5NS, $D_{10}W$, and $^1/_2NS$

Compatible drugs

Limited data available

Incompatible drugs

Diltiazem HCl (5 mg/mL)

ACYCLOVIR SODIUM
Zovirax®, Glaxo Wellcome Inc.

Method of administration
Intermittent intravenous infusion (over 1 hour) and *not* by direct intravenous, intramuscular, or subcutaneous injection

Dosing and administration
Standard: 500 mg or 1 g/250 mL of D_5W (no more than 7 mg/mL)

Acyclovir is active against various Herpesviridae, including herpes simplex virus types 1 and 2 (HSV-1, HSV-2), varicella-zoster, herpesvirus simiae (B virus), and cytomegalovirus.

For both mucosal and cutaneous herpes simplex (HSV-1 and HSV-2) infections in immunocompromised patients: Administer 5 mg/kg every 8 hours (15 mg/kg/day) intravenously for 5 to 14 days until the lesions have resolved satisfactorily.

Severe initial clinical episodes of herpes genitalis: Administer the same dose as above for 5 to 7 days, up to 21 days until resolution of lesions is satisfactory.

Herpes simplex encephalitis: Administer 10 mg/kg intravenously every 8 hours (30 mg/kg/day) for 10 to 21 days of treatment, depending on the patient's condition.

Varicella or herpes zoster in immunocompromised patients: Administer 7.5 mg to 10 mg/kg every 8 hours (22.5 to 30 mg/kg/day) intravenously for 7 to 14 days.

Bone marrow transplant recipients: Administer 5 mg/kg every 8 hours (if HSV seropositive) to every 12 hours (if clinical symptoms of herpes simplex) or 10 mg/kg every 8 hours in patients who are cytomegalovirus seropositive.

General

Doses should be based on the smaller of either ideal or actual body weight.

The patient needs to be adequately hydrated to decrease risk of nephrotoxicity secondary to precipitation of acyclovir crystals in renal tubules.

Dose or interval adjustment is required for patients with renal insufficiency (creatinine clearance less than 50 mL/minute). For patients with a creatinine clearance of 25 to 50 mL/minute, increase the interval to every 12 hours. For a creatinine clearance less than 25 mL/minute, increase the interval to every 24 hours. Administer the medication after hemodialysis, if the drug is not administered immediately after hemodialysis, then administer 60% of the dose as a supplement. No dosage adjustment required for hepatic failure.

Acyclovir should be used during pregnancy only when the potential benefits justify the possible risks to the fetus. The drug's potential for producing chromosomal damage should be considered.

Monitor
Signs of infection (temperature, white blood cell count with differential), hydration status (urine output), serum creatinine, blood urea nitrogen, signs of nephrotoxicity (pre-existing renal failure and dehydration increase risk), liver enzymes, inflammation or phlebitis at injection site (concentrations less than 10 mg/mL increase risk), nausea, and central nervous system effects (eg, tremors, seizures, confusion, lethargy; higher incidence with doses more than 10 mg/kg/day or in patients with underlying neurologic or renal disease).

Protect from light: no

Special considerations: none

pH: approximately 11

Stability
Reconstituted solutions remain stable for 24 hours (12 hours in reconstituted vial) at room temperature; may precipitate if refrigerated.

Solution compatibility: D_5W, NS, D_5NS, and LR

Compatible drugs

Allopurinol sodium
Amikacin sulfate
Ampicillin sodium
Cefamandole nafate
Cefazolin sodium
Cefoperazone sodium
Ceforanide sodium
Cefotaxime sodium
Cefoxitin sodium
Ceftazidime sodium
Ceftizoxime sodium
Ceftriaxone sodium
Cefuroxime sodium
Chloramphenicol sodium-succinate
Cimetidine HCl
Clindamycin phosphate
Dexamethasone sodium phosphate
Diltiazem HCl (≤1 mg/mL)
Diphenhydramine HCl
Doxycycline hyclate
Erythromycin lactobionate
Fluconazole
Gentamycin sulfate
Heparin sodium
Hydrocortisone sodium
Hydromorphone HCl
Imipenem-cilastatin
Lorazepam
Magnesium sulfate
Melphalan HCl
Meperidine HCl
Methylprednisolone sodium succinate
Metoclopramide HCl
Metronidazole
Nafcillin sodium
Oxacillin sodium
Paclitaxel
Penicillin G potassium
Pentobarbital
Perphenazine
Piperacillin sodium
Potassium chloride
Ranitidine HCl
Sodium bicarbonate
Tacrolimus
Ticarcillin disodium
Tobramycin sulfate
Trimethoprim-sulfameth-oxazole
Vancomycin HCl

Incompatible drugs

Amsacrine
Aztreonam
Cefepime HCl
Diltiazem HCl (>1 mg/mL)
Dobutamine HCl
Dopamine HCl
Fludarabine phosphate
Foscarnet sodium
Idarubicin HCl
Meropenem
Morphine sulfate
Ondansetron HCl
Piperacillin sodium tazobac-tam sodium
Sargramostim
Vinorelbine tartrate

ADENOSINE
Adenocard®, Fujisawa USA, Inc.

Method of administration
Direct intravenous injection

Dosing and administration
Standard: 6 mg/2 mL (no further dilution required)

Treatment and diagnosis of paroxysmal supraventricular tachycardia (including PSVT associated with Wolff-Parkinson-White syndrome)

Initiate therapy with 6 mg given as a direct intravenous injection (administered over a 1- to 2-second period). *Administer either directly into an antecubital vein or, if through an intravenous catheter, administer as proximally as possible and flush the line with 20 mL NS. If the first dose does not result in elimination of the supraventricular tachycardia within 1 to 2 minutes, 12 mg should be given as a rapid, direct intravenous injection. The 12-mg dose can be repeated if necessary. Doses larger than 12 mg as a single injection are not recommended. If patient has not responded to a cumulative dose of 30 mg, the diagnosis should be reevaluated.

Adenosine has been used as a continuous infusion in NS for management of pulmonary hypertension in emergent situations to control hypertension and to decrease cardiac afterload.

The effects of adenosine are antagonized by methylxanthines (eg, theophylline, caffeine). Larger doses of adenosine may be required or the drug may be ineffective.

The effects of adenosine may be accentuated by dipyridamole, and lower doses of adenosine may be required.

Monitor
ECG resolution of dysrhythmias (to assess effectiveness; dysrhythmias occur in 55% of patients; a brief period of asystole [15 seconds] may occur), heart rate, blood pressure, respiratory status (eg, bronchospasm and dyspnea, especially in patients

with a history of asthma, usually resolve within a few minutes of administration), facial flushing, anxiety, and chest pressure/pain.

Protect from light: no

Special consideration: none

pH: 5.5 to 7.5

Stability: do not refrigerate; precipitation may occur

Solution compatibility: NS

Drug compatibility: limited data available

*A lower initial dose (1 to 3 mg) can be given if injected through a central venous line.

ALBUMIN, HUMAN
various manufacturers

Method of administration
Intermittent intravenous infusion

Dosing and administration
Standard: 50 mg/mL and 250 mg/mL

Treatment of hemorrhagic and nonhemorrhagic shock
For acute therapy, administer 500 mL of albumin 5%. If inadequate response in 30 minutes, administer an additional 500 mL. Dose and duration of treatment should be based on blood pressure, degree of shock, hemoglobin, hematocrit, and patient response.

The rate of administration for treatment of shock should be as quickly as possible, but once the plasma volume approaches normality, the rate of the 5% solution should not exceed 2 to 4 mL/minute, and the rate of the 25% solution should not exceed 1 mL/minute.

Crystalloids (eg, lactated Ringer's solution and 0.9% sodium chloride) are generally considered first-line therapy for treatment of hemorrhagic and nonhemorrhagic shock because crystalloids and colloids are equally effective and crystalloids are less expensive. Colloids should be considered in patients not adequately responding (hemodynamically unstable) to crystalloid solutions.

Treatment of hypoproteinemia
The administration of albumin as a nutrient in the treatment of chronic hypoalbuminemia is generally not recommended. In acute hypoalbuminemic states, a 5% albumin solution has been used and dosed based on target serum albumin concentrations. Different concentrations have been used as endpoints, but are generally in the range of 2.5 g/dL or 3.0 g/dL. In one study, however, there was no difference in mortality, complication rate, length of time in an intensive care unit or total days in hospital, duration of ventilatory dependence, or duration of

parenteral feeding compared with patients who did not receive albumin.

Solutions containing 5% albumin are generally used in hypovolemic patients, with more concentrated solutions used in patients with a low serum sodium who are fluid restricted.

General

No more than 250 g of albumin (5% or 25%) should be administered within a 48-hour period. If used for treatment of shock, consider administration of whole blood or plasma in these patients.

The hypertonic solution (25%) draws 3.5 times its own volume into the intravascular space from the interstitial compartment.

Use caution in patients with renal or hepatic insufficiency because of an increase in protein load and an increase in oncotic pressure.

Conditions in which albumin has been used include cardiac surgery (cardiopulmonary bypass pump), cerebral edema, cirrhosis, renal and liver transplant, hepatic resection, acute nephrotic syndrome, plasmaphoresis (in conjunction with large-volume exchange), severe necrotizing pancreatitis, and thermal injury.

Monitor

Signs and symptoms of shock, including blood pressure (hypotension), heart rate (tachycardia), respirations (hyperventilation), central nervous system effects (agitation to coma), fluid status (urine output of less than 20 mL/hour), acid/base status (lactic acidosis), and cold, clammy skin.

Other monitoring parameters: Chills, fever, nausea, vomiting, and, blood pressure (hypotension) may occur from too rapid an infusion. Rapid infusion may also result in vascular overload (signs include pulmonary edema or cardiac failure).

Protect from light: no

Special considerations: none

pH: 6.9 ± 0.5

Stability

Do not use if the solution is turbid or contains deposits; use within 4 hours after opening the vial. Administration needs to be complete within 6 hours after opening the container. Solution can be stored at room temperature.

Solution compatibility: D_5W, NS, $D_{10}W$, LR, $^1/_2$NS, and D_5NS

Compatible drugs

Diltiazem HCl

Incompatible drugs

Vancomycin HCl
Verapamil HCl

ALTEPLASE, t-PA
Activase®, Genentech, Inc.

Methods of administration
Intermittent intravenous injection and also administered by intracoronary or intra-arterial routes

Dosing and administration
Standard: 100 mg/200 mL of NS

Coronary artery thrombi and acute pulmonary embolus
The recommended dose is based upon patient weight, not to exceed a total dose of 100 mg. For patients weighing more than 67 kg, the recommended dose is 100 mg as a 15-mg intravenous bolus, followed by 50 mg infused over the next 30 minutes, and then 35 mg infused over the next 60 minutes. For patients weighing 67 kg or less, the recommended dose is 15 mg as an intravenous bolus, followed by 0.75 mg/kg (not to exceed 50 mg) infused over the next 30 minutes, and then 0.50 mg/kg (not to exceed 35 mg) over the next 60 minutes.

Monitor
Indication of reperfusion: documented by coronary angiography (infarct artery open), reduction of ST segment elevation (may see initial reperfusion dysrhythmias), resolution of chest pain (may have initial exacerbation of chest pain), and echocardiography (improvement in regional wall motion).

Other monitoring parameters include: (1) bleeding (eg, external bleeding around venipuncture sites, hypotension, hematuria, abdominal pain, sudden change in mental status such as that seen with a CNS bleed, hematochezia, bleeding from hemorrhoids, and blurred vision), (2) heart rate, (3) extravasation (causes ecchymosis or inflammation) and (4) aPTT.

Protect from light: yes (does not affect potency of reconstituted solutions)

Special considerations: none

pH: approximately 7.3

Stability
Refrigerate; must be used within 8 hours of reconstitution; pale yellow in color upon reconstitution. Reconstitute immediately before use. Stable in pH range of 5 to 7.5. Diluents other than sterile water for injection without preservatives should not be used for reconstitution. Do not use solutions containing preservatives.

Solution compatibility: D_5W (dilution lower than 0.5 mg/mL solution may result in precipitation) and NS

Compatible drugs
Lidocaine HCl
Metoprolol tartrate
Propranolol HCl

Incompatible drugs
Dobutamine HCl
Dopamine HCl
Heparin sodium
Nitroglycerin

AMIKACIN SULFATE
Amikin®, Apothecon, and other manufacturers

Methods of administration
Intramuscular, intermittent intravenous infusion (over 30 minutes), intrathecal, and intraventricular

Dosing and administration
Standard: 500 mg/100 mL of D_5W or NS

Amikacin is an aminoglycoside antibiotic that is active against many aerobic gram-negative bacteria, including *Acinetobacter calcoaceticus, Escherichia coli, Haemophilus influenzae, Moraxella lacunata, Neisseria* sp, *Proteus* sp, *Serratia* sp, and *Pseudomonas* sp (including most strains of *Pseudomonas aeruginosa*). Amikacin is active against some strains of bacteria, especially *Proteus* sp, *Pseudomonas* sp, and *Serratia* sp, that are not susceptible to other aminoglycosides. Amikacin is active against some aerobic gram-positive bacteria, including *Staphylococcus aureus* and *Staphylococcus epidermidis*. Amikacin is only minimally active against streptococci.

Treatment of suspected or documented gram-negative infections generally resistant to gentamicin or tobramycin
Administer a loading dose of 7.5 mg/kg, then 15 mg/kg daily in two or three divided doses. Dosage should be based on total body weight (TBW) and not ideal body weight (IBW), unless patient is morbidly obese. A typical dose for patients with adequate renal function (less than 70 mL/minute) is 7.5 mg/kg every 8 hours. If patient is morbidly obese, then weight should be determined by using the formula IBW + 0.4 (TBW − IBW). Treatment typically continues for 7 to 10 days.

Once-a-day aminoglycoside regimens are also used but have not been widely studied in intensive care unit patients. A dose of 15 to 20 mg/kg is administered to patients who have an estimated creatinine clearance of at least 60 mL/minute. Patients with compromised renal function require that the interval be adjusted according to pharmacokinetic parameters to achieve a trough of less than 5 μg/mL.

Intrathecal administration
Administer 4 to 20 mg for treatment of gram-negative bacillary meningitis. Typically given concurrently with systemic therapy.

General
Dosage or interval needs to be adjusted in patients with renal insufficiency (95% of drug excreted unchanged through the kidneys). For a creatinine clearance of 50 to 70 mL/minute, increase the interval to every 12 hours; for a creatinine clearance of 30 to 50 mL/minute, give every 18 hours. For a creatinine clearance of 15 to 30 mL/minute, give every 24 hours. For a creatinine clearance of less than 15 mL/minute, give initial dose × 1 and then dose when random level is less than 5.0 μg/mL.

Obtain amikacin serum levels to determine appropriate dose and regimen. Amikacin is approximately 50% dialyzable. Administer dose following hemodialysis. No change required in patients with hepatic failure.

Monitor
Signs of infection (temperature, white blood cell count with differential), culture and susceptibility, signs of nephrotoxicity (serum creatinine, blood urea nitrogen, fluid status), signs of ototoxicity (auditory and vestibular toxicity, tinnitus, vertigo), and serum amikacin concentrations.

The risk of nephrotoxicity is dependent on several factors,

Therapeutic drug monitoring considerations
   Sample collection when patient is at steady state:
      Peak: 30 minutes after end of 30-minute infusion
               60 minutes after intramuscular injection
      Trough: within 30 minutes prior to dose
   Therapeutic range:
      Peak: 20 to 30 μg/mL
      Trough: 3 to 8 μg/mL

---

including concomitant nephrotoxic drugs, prolonged elevated trough concentrations, age, hydration status, dose, and duration of treatment. Generally reversible upon discontinuation of the medication.

Protect from light: no

Special considerations
If concomitant penicillin use is needed, administer at least 1 hour from the amikacin and flush tubing prior to administration. Precipitation has occurred when amikacin sulfate is administered through a heparinized intravenous cannula. Flush with NS before and after administering drugs.

pH: 3.5 to 5.5

Stability
Stable for 24 hours at room temperature and for 2 days if refrigerated.

Solution compatibility: D_5W, NS, $D_5\frac{1}{2}NS$, $D_{10}W$, and LR

Compatible drugs

Acyclovir sodium	Idarubicin HCl
Amiodarone HCl	IL-2
Amsacrine	Labetalol HCl
Aztreonam	Magnesium sulfate
Cyclophosphamide	Melphalan HCl
Cyclosporine	Meperidine
Diltiazem HCl	Morphine sulfate
Enalaprilat	Ondansetron HCl
Esmolol HCl	Oxytocin
Filgrastim	Paclitaxel
Fluconazole	Perphenazine
Fludarabine phosphate	Sargramostim
Foscarnet sodium	Teniposide
Furosemide	Vinorelbine tartrate
Hydromorphone	Zidovudine

Incompatible drugs

Allopurinol sodium
Aminophylline
Amphotericin B
Ampicillin sodium
Azathioprine sodium
Azlocillin
Cefazolin sodium
Cefoperazone
Folic acid
Ganciclovir sodium
Heparin sodium
Hetastarch
Methicillin sodium
Pentamidine isethionate
Pentobarbital sodium
Phenytoin sodium
Propofol
Warfarin sodium

AMINOPHYLLINE
various manufacturers

Methods of administration
Intermittent intravenous infusion (do not infuse at a rate exceeding 20 mg/minute), continuous intravenous infusion, and *not* intramuscular (pain on injection)

Dosing and administration
Standard: 500 mg/500 mL of D_5W or NS (maximum concentration: 1000 mg/250 mL)

Pulmonary diseases associated with bronchospasm or to stimulate diaphragmatic contractility in patients on ventilators
Administer 5 to 6 mg/kg (300 mg to 600 mg in 50 or 100 mL of D_5W or NS) infused over 30 minutes, followed by a continuous intravenous infusion. Aminophylline infusion rate should be based on the following parameters:

Adults (smoking)	0.7 mg/kg/hour
Adults (nonsmoking)	0.5 mg/kg/hour
Congestive heart failure, cor pulmonale, or liver disease	0.25 mg/kg/hour

Infusion rates are designed to be used with ideal body weight for obese individuals and to achieve a target serum theophylline concentration of 10 µg/mL. Continuous infusion rate typically ranges from 20 to 50 mg/hour. If patient is currently maintained on aminophylline and the patient's theophylline blood levels are subtherapeutic, administer 1.0 mg/kg aminophylline for every 2 µg/mL increase in serum theophylline concentration desired.

To switch to oral therapy, the infusion is discontinued 2 hours after sustained release dose is given. The daily dose of aminophylline should be multiplied by a factor of 0.8 to determine the dose of theophylline necessary; round to the nearest 50 mg. When switching to oral theophylline, multiply the hourly continuous infusion rate by 10 and give that dose every 12 hours.

For example: (30 mg/hour) (10) = 300 mg; give the patient 300 mg every 12 hours.

$$1 \text{ g aminophylline} = 0.8 \text{ g theophylline}$$

Monitor

Resolution of bronchospasm, increased movement of air, decreased wheezing, hydration status (diuretic effect of theophylline), blood pressure (hypotension, especially if medication is given too quickly; avoid loading rate greater than 20 mg/minute), and measure serum drug concentrations.

Signs of toxicity include nausea, vomiting, tachycardia, agitation, seizures (many times refractory to standard therapy), and arrhythmias.

Co-administration of medications such as cimetidine, ciprofloxacin, diltiazem, clarithromycin, fluconazole, and erythromycin may decrease theophylline clearance (increasing theophylline serum concentration). Cigarette smoking, phenytoin, rifampin, phenobarbital, and carbamazepine may increase theophylline clearance, resulting in lower serum drug levels.

Therapeutic drug monitoring considerations
> Sample collection:
>> For continuous infusion, take a single level more than 24 hours after start of infusion or after dosage adjustment.
>> For intermittent infusion, take a trough level within 60 minutes prior to dose.
> Therapeutic range:
>> 10 to 20 µg/mL

Protect from light: yes, if infusion of solution requires more than 24 hours (degradation only after extended periods of time, eg, more than 8 weeks)

Special considerations: none

pH: 8.6 to 9.0

Stability

Maintains stability at pH of 8; precipitation occurs at pH <8; stable at room temperature for at least 24 hours after dilution.

Solution compatibility: D_5W, NS, LR, D_5NS, $D_{10}W$, and ½NS

Compatible drugs

Amrinone lactate	Meropenem
Atracurium besylate	Morphine sulfate
Aztreonam	Pancuronium bromide
Cimetidine HCl	Piperacillin sodium-tazobac-
Enalaprilat	tam sodium
Esmolol HCl	Potassium chloride
Filgrastim	Sargramostim
Fluconazole	Ranitidine HCl
Foscarnet sodium	Tacrolimus
Famotidine	Vecuronium bromide
Labetalol HCl	

Incompatible drugs

Amikacin sulfate	Isoproterenol HCl
Amiodarone HCl	Magnesium sulfate
Ampicillin sodium	Meperidine HCl
Ascorbic acid	Methadone HCl
Cefepime HCl	Midazolam HCl
Ceftriaxone sodium	Minocycline HCl
Chlorpromazine HCl	Norepinephrine bitartrate
Ciprofloxacin	Ondansetron HCl
Clindamycin phosphate	Penicillin G potassium
Codeine phosphate	Penicillin G sodium
Diltiazem HCl	Phenytoin sodium
Diphenhydramine HCl	Pentamidine isethionate
Dobutamine HCl	Prochlorperazine edisylate
Epinephrine HCl	Promethazine HCl
Ganciclovir sodium	Propofol
Haloperidol lactate	Quinidine gluconate
Hydroxyzine HCl	Vancomycin HCl
Hydralazine HCl	Verapamil HCl
Imipenem-cilastatin sodium	Warfarin sodium
Insulin, regular	

AMIODARONE HYDROCHLORIDE
Cordarone®, Wyeth-Ayerst Laboratories

Methods of administration
Intermittent and continuous intravenous infusion

Dosing and administration
Standard: 150 mg/100 mL of D_5W

Life-threatening ventricular arrhythmias or supraventricular arrhythmias

There are several methods by which amiodarone may be given. One method is to administer the medication in a three-phase sequence: rapid loading dose, slow infusion, and maintenance dose. Administer 150 mg in 10 mL D_5W over the first 10 minutes (15 mg/minute). Then 360 mg is administered over the next 6 hours (1 mg/minute) followed by a maintenance infusion of 540 mg over the remaining 18 hours (0.5 mg/minute).

After the first 24 hours, a maintenance infusion of 0.5 mg/minute (concentration of 1 to 6 mg/mL; 720 mg/24 hours) can be initiated. In the event of breakthrough episodes of ventricular fibrillation or hemodynamically unstable ventricular tachycardia, supplemental infusions of amiodarone 150 mg may be administered over 10 minutes.

Most patients may require therapy for 48 to 96 hours; however, infusions of 0.5 mg/minute for up to 2 to 3 weeks have been used. Limited data are available describing intravenous use in patients for a longer time.

Alternative loading strategies include 5 mg/kg over 20 minutes for supraventricular tachycardia, followed by an infusion of 10 mg/kg/day.

Monitor
ECG resolution of arrhythmia (amiodarone can also cause an arrhythmia [eg, AV block]), and blood pressure (hypotension, especially with too rapid an infusion secondary to polysorbate 80 as a solubilizing agent).

If long-term therapy is anticipated, liver function tests, pulmonary function tests, and thyroid function tests are suggested as baseline prior to institution, and a slit lamp evaluation at 6 months.

Amiodarone inhibits the metabolism of digoxin, quinidine, lidocaine, procainamide, warfarin, and cyclosporine, which may result in increased effects of these medications. Concomitant administration of phenytoin and cimetidine may increase the effects of amiodarone.

Protect from light: yes (not necessary during administration)

Special considerations
Administer by volumetric infusion pump with an in line-filter. Amiodarone infusions that exceed 2 hours must be administered in glass or polyolefin containers. PVC tubing, however, can be used. Solutions containing a concentration of 2 mg/mL or more should be administered via a central venous catheter.

pH: approximately 4

Stability
A concentration less than 0.6 mg/mL in D_5W is unstable. Data on compatibility with NS are conflicting.

Solution compatibility: D_5W

Compatible drugs

Amikacin sulfate	Isoproterenol HCl
Bretylium tosylate	Labetalol HCl
Cefazolin sodium	Lidocaine HCl
Clindamycin phosphate	Metaraminol bitartrate
Dobutamine HCl	Metronidazole HCl
Dopamine HCl	Midazolam HCl
Doxycycline hyclate	Morphine sulfate
Erythromycin lactobionate	Nitroglycerin
Esmolol HCl	Norepinephrine bitartrate
Gentamicin sulfate	Penicillin G potassium
Insulin, regular	Phentolamine mesylate

Compatible drugs continued

Phenylephrine HCl
Potassium chloride
Procainamide HCl
Tobramycin sulfate
Vancomycin HCl

Incompatible drugs

Aminophylline
Cefamandole nafate
Cefazolin sodium
Heparin sodium
Mezlocillin sodium
Quinidine gluconate
Sodium bicarbonate

AMPHOTERICIN B
Fungizone®, Apothecon, and other manufacturers

Methods of administration
Intermittent intravenous infusion (over 1 to 4 hours), and other routes such as intrathecal, intrapleural, and intra-articular

Dosing and administration
Standard: 50 mg/500 mL of D_5W (maximum concentration of 0.1 mg/mL for peripheral administration and 1 mg/mL for central administration)

Amphotericin B is an antifungal agent that usually inhibits the following fungi: *Candida* sp, *Aspergillus fumigatus, Coccidioides immitis, Cryptococcus neoformans, Histoplasma capsulatum,* and *Sporothrix schenckii. Blastomyces dermatitidis* may require slightly higher drug concentrations for inhibition. Amphotericin B is active against the following protozoa: *Leishmania braziliensis, L mexicana,* and *L tropica.*

Treatment of severe systemic infections and meningitis (eg, Cryptococcus*, blastomycosis and histoplasmosis)*
A test dose of 1 mg infused over 30 to 60 minutes is recommended by the manufacturer, but may not be necessary. Monitor for signs of an anaphylactic reaction (eg, patient's heart rate, respiratory rate, and blood pressure) for 4 hours. If no significant adverse reactions, initiate therapy with a daily dose of 0.25 mg/kg to 0.3 mg/kg of body weight over 1 to 4 hours. The dose is gradually increased on subsequent days by 0.25 mg/kg as tolerated until the desired daily dose of 0.5 to 1 mg/kg is achieved. It is generally not recommended to exceed 1.5 mg/kg/dose. For treatment of disseminated candidiasis, coccidioidomycosis, and aspergillosis, the usual intravenous dose is 0.5 mg/kg to 1 mg/kg daily, although higher dosages have been used in rapidly progressing infections.

The cumulative dose and duration of treatment depend on the type and severity of infection; the dose is generally 1 to 4 g.

Intrathecal administration
Initiate therapy with a dose of 25 µg every 48 to 72 hours, and increase the dose until a maximum is reached without causing discomfort. Typical doses are 0.3 to 1 mg administered intrathecally every 48 to 72 hours depending on type and severity of infection.

General
Fever and chills are common infusion-related side effects of amphotericin B. To help prevent the occurrence or severity of the reaction, consider premedicating the patient 30 minutes prior to the dose as follows: Use acetaminophen (325 mg to 650 mg orally or rectally) and diphenhydramine (25 to 50 mg orally or intravenously) for fever and myalgias; hydrocortisone (50 mg intravenously) for fever and chills; or meperidine (50 mg intravenously) for shaking chills (rigors) that are refractory to hydrocortisone.

Dose or frequency adjustment is not required for patients with renal dysfunction. However, if symptoms of renal toxicity occur, the total daily dose can be decreased by 50% or given every other day. Amphotericin B is not removed by hemodialysis. No dosage changes required for hepatic failure.

Three new lipid formulations of amphotericin B are currently available (Abelcet®, Amphotec®, and AmBisome®). Abelcet® and AmBisome® are both an amphotericin B lipid complex. Amphotec® is a colloidal dispersion of amphotericin B. All three products are generally reserved for the treatment of fungal infections in patients who are refractory to or intolerant of conventional amphotericin B therapy. Patients with renal insufficiency (less than 2.0 mg/dL) have experienced a decline in serum creatinine at a lower rate than with the traditional formulation. The medications can be given in the following doses:

• Abelcet®: Recommended daily dosage is 5 mg/kg given as a single infusion

• Amphotec®: Initial recommended daily dosage is 3 to 4 mg/kg. Dose may be increased to 6 mg/kg/day if there is no improvement or evidence of progression of disease.

• AmBisome®: The recommended initial dose for empirical therapy is 3.0 mg/kg/day and for systemic fungal infections caused by *Aspergillus* sp, *Candida* sp, and *Cryptococcus* sp, it is 3.0 to 5.0 mg/kg/day.

The information in this monograph refers only to the traditional formulation of amphotericin B.

Monitor

Signs of infection (temperature, white blood cell count with differential), potassium, magnesium (hypomagnesemia), BUN, serum creatinine, and urine output, hydration, fever, chills, liver function tests, and phlebitis and pain at injection site. Rapid intravenous injection has resulted in hypotension and arrhythmias. Infusion-related adverse events include headache, malaise, generalized pain, anorexia, hypertension or hypotension, flushing, nausea, and vomiting. Amphotericin increases serum concentration of cyclosporine.

Nephrotoxicity is generally reversible unless there is underlying disease or a cumulative dose exceeding 3 to 4 g. An increased risk of nephrotoxicity exists with concomitant administration of nephrotoxic drugs (eg, aminoglycosides). Risk may be decreased by increasing the sodium load via saline bolusing (500 mL NS over 30 minutes) prior to the dose.

Hypokalemia may occur secondary to renal tubular excretion of potassium; administration of corticosteroids may potentiate this effect. Monitor for signs and symptoms of hypokalemia, including muscle weakness.

Protect from light: yes; exposure (<24 hours) does affect potency

Special considerations

Reconstitute with sterile water without preservatives, not bacteriostatic water. If an in-line filter is used, the mean pore diameter must be 1 micron or greater.

pH: 5.7 to 8

Stability

pH range for stability is 6 to 7 with turbidity occurring at a pH <6.

Solution compatibility: D_5W, $D_{10}W$, *not* stable in NS, D_5NS, or LR

Compatible drugs (in D_5W)

Diltiazem HCl
Tacrolimus

Incompatible drugs

Amikacin sulfate
Amrinone lactate
Atracurium besylate
Atropine sulfate
Aztreonam
Bretylium tosylate
Bumetanide
Butorphanol tartrate
Calcium chloride
Calcium gluconate
Cefepime HCl
Cefmetazole sodium
Cefotetan disodium
Ceftizoxime sodium
Chlorpromazine HCl
Cimetidine HCl
Clindamycin phosphate
Dexamethasone sodium
  phosphate
Digoxin
Diphenhydramine HCl
Dobutamine HCl
Dopamine HCl
Doxycycline hyclate
Enalaprilat
Ephedrine sulfate
Epinephrine HCl
Epoetin alfa
Erythromycin lactobionate
Esmolol HCl

Famotidine
Filgrastim
Fluconazole
Ganciclovir sodium
Gentamicin sulfate
Haloperidol lactate
Hydrocortisone sodium
  succinate
Hydroxyzine HCl
Isoproterenol HCl
Ketorolac tromethamine
Labetalol HCl
Lidocaine HCl
Magnesium sulfate
Meperidine HCl
Methylprednisolone
  sodium succinate
Metoclopramide HCl
Metoprolol tartrate
Metronidazole HCl
Midazolam HCl
Minocycline HCl
Morphine sulfate
Nafcillin sodium
Nalbuphine HCl
Nitroprusside sodium
Norepinephrine bitartrate
Ondansetron HCl
Paclitaxel
Penicillin G potassium

Penicillin G sodium
Pentamidine isethionate
Pentazocine lactate
Phentolamine mesylate
Phenylephrine HCl
Piperacillin sodium
Piperacillin sodium tazobac-
    tam sodium
Potassium chloride
Prochlorperazine edisylate
Promethazine HCl
Propranolol HCl
Protamine sulfate
Pyridoxine HCl
Quinidine gluconate
Ranitidine HCl
Ritodrine HCl
Sodium bicarbonate
Succinylcholine chloride
Thiamine HCl
Tobramycin sulfate
Urokinase
Vancomycin HCl
Vasopressin
Verapamil HCl

Methods of administration

Intramuscular, direct intravenous injection (over 3 to 5 minutes if up to 500 mg and 10 to 15 minutes for larger doses; administer into a vein or into the tubing of freely flowing compatible intravenous solution), and intermittent intravenous infusion (over 20 to 30 minutes)

Dosing and administration

Standard: 500 mg to 1 g/50 mL and 2 g/100 mL of NS (concentrated solutions of 60 mg/mL)

Ampicillin is an aminopenicillin that is active against many gram-positive aerobic cocci including nonpenicillinase-producing strains of *Staphylococcus aureus* and *Staphylococcus epidermidis*; group A, B, C, and G streptococci; *Streptococcus pneumoniae*, viridans streptococci; and some strains of enterococci. It is also active against several gram-positive aerobic bacilli (*Corynebacterium diphtheriae, Listeria monocytogenes,* and *Bacillus anthracis*). Ampicillin is active against some gram-negative aerobic bacteria (*Neisseria meningitidis*; nonpenicillinase-producing *Neisseria gonorrhoeae*; *Haemophilus influenzae* and some strains of *Haemophilus parainfluenzae*; some strains of *Escherichia coli*, *Proteus mirabilis, Salmonella* sp, and *Shigella* sp; *Bordetella pertussis,* and *Eikenella corrodens*).

For treatment of infections: respiratory tract, soft tissue, urinary tract, intra-abdominal, and gonococcal
Administer 500 mg to 1.5 g intramuscularly every 4 to 6 hours. For intermittent intravenous infusion, administer 500 mg to 2 g every 6 hours.

Treatment of bacterial endocarditis or enterococcal bacteremia
Administer 2 g every 4 hours. Use gentamicin with ampicillin for synergy.

*Prevention of bacterial endocarditis for genitourinary/
gastrointestinal procedures*

Administer 2 g ampicillin sodium plus gentamicin 1.5 mg/kg
not to exceed 120 mg, either intravenously or intramuscularly
30 minutes prior to procedure, followed by 1.0 g amoxicillin 6
hours after initial dose, or repeat parenteral dose 8 hours after
initial dose.

General

Dosage or interval adjustment required for renal insufficiency.
For a creatinine clearance of 10 to 30 mL/minute, increase the
interval to every 6 to 8 hours. For creatinine clearance less than
10 mL/minute, extend the interval to 8 to 12 hours. For
patients receiving hemodialysis, either give a maintenance
dose after dialysis or give an additional 500 mg after dialysis
if the regular dose was administered prior to dialysis. No
dosage adjustment required for hepatic failure.

Monitor

Signs of infection (temperature, white blood cell count with
differential), culture and susceptibility, serum creatinine, blood
urea nitrogen, fluid status (input and output), diarrhea, hypersensitivity reactions, and signs of central nervous system toxicity (neuromuscular hyperirritability and convulsions).

Ampicillin is contraindicated for use in patients with a
severe, documented allergy to penicillin antibiotics. Ampicillin
should be used cautiously in patients with allergies to
cephalosporins or carbapenems (eg, imipenem) as cross-reactivity may exist. Cross-reactivity occurs with cephalosporins
in 3% to 15% of patients.

Protect from light: no

Special considerations

If concomitant aminoglycoside use is needed, administer at
least 1 hour from the ampicillin and flush tubing prior to
administration.

pH: 8 to 10 (reconstituted solutions containing 10 mg/mL)

Stability

Stable in NS for 8 hours at room temperature (2 days if refrigerated); limited stability in D_5W (2 hours); intramuscular or medication prepared for direct intravenous injection should be used within 1 hour of reconstitution.

Solution compatibility: NS (preferred)

Compatible drugs (in NS)

Acyclovir sodium	Insulin, regular
Allopurinol sodium	Labetalol HCl
Aztreonam	Magnesium sulfate
Calcium gluconate	Melphalan HCl
Cyclophosphamide	Meperidine HCl
Cyclosporine	Morphine sulfate
Enalaprilat	Ofloxacin
Esmolol HCl	Perphenazine
Famotidine	Phytonadione
Filgrastim	Potassium chloride
Fludarabine phosphate	Tacrolimus
Foscarnet sodium	Teniposide
Heparin sodium	Tolazoline HCl
Hydromorphone HCl	

Incompatible drugs

Amikacin sulfate	Ganciclovir sodium
Aminophylline	Gentamicin sulfate
Amrinone lactate	Hetastarch
Buprenorphine HCl	Hydralazine
Chlorpromazine	Hydrocortisone
Diltiazem HCl	Hydroxyzine HCl
Diphenhydramine HCl	Lidocaine HCl
Dobutamine HCl	Methylprednisolone sodium
Dopamine HCl	succinate
Doxycycline hyclate	Metoclopramide HCl
Epinephrine HCl	Midazolam HCl
Erythromycin lactobionate	Minocycline HCl
Fluconazole	Ondansetron HCl

Pentamidine isethionate
Pentazocine lactate
Pentobarbital sodium
Phenobarbital sodium
Prochlorperazine edisylate
Promethazine HCl
Propofol

Protamine sulfate
Quinidine gluconate
Sargramostim
Sodium bicarbonate
Verapamil HCl
Vinorelbine tartrate

AMPICILLIN SODIUM-SULBACTAM SODIUM
Unasyn®, Pfizer Inc

Methods of administration
Intramuscular, direct intravenous injection (over 10 to 15 minutes; administer into a vein or into the tubing of freely flowing compatible intravenous solution), and intermittent intravenous infusion (over 15 to 30 minutes)

Dosing and administration
Standard: 1.5 g/50 mL or 3 g/100 mL of NS

Ampicillin sodium-sulbactam sodium is an aminopenicillin plus a b-lactamase inhibitor that has a wide spectrum of activity against many gram-positive and gram-negative aerobic and anaerobic bacteria. Ampicillin sodium-sulbactam is active against organisms susceptible to ampicillin alone (see ampicillin). In addition, because sulbactam can inhibit certain b-lactamases that generally inactivate ampicillin, ampicillin sodium-sulbactam is active against many b-lactamase-producing organisms that are resistant to ampicillin alone, including ampicillin-resistant strains of staphylococci, *Haemophilus* sp, *Neisseria* sp, and *Bacteroides* sp.

For treatment of the following infections: skin and skin structure, intra-abdominal, ischemic/diabetic foot, urinary tract, polymicrobial upper and lower respiratory tract, and gynecological or pelvic
Administer ampicillin sodium-sulbactam in doses of 1.5 to 3 g every 6 hours. The total dose of sulbactam should not exceed 4 g per day.

1.5 g of Unasyn® = 1 g ampicillin plus 0.5 g sulbactam as the sodium salt

3.0 g of Unasyn® = 2 g ampicillin plus 1 g sulbactam as the sodium salt

Dosage or frequency adjustment is required for patients with renal insufficiency. In patients with a creatinine clearance of 10 to 30 mL/minute, administer 100% of dose every 8 to 12 hours. In patients with a creatinine clearance of less than 10 mL/minute, administer every 12 to 24 hours. For patients receiving hemodialysis no supplement is required if the maintenance dose is administered after dialysis. No dosage adjustment is required for hepatic failure.

Monitor
Signs of infection (temperature, white blood cell count with differential), culture and susceptibility, hypersensitivity reactions, diarrhea, and signs of central nervous system toxicity (neuromuscular irritability and convulsions).

Ampicillin sodium-sulbactam is contraindicated in patients with severe, documented allergy to penicillin antibiotics. Ampicillin should be cautiously used in patients with allergies to cephalosporins as cross-reactivity may exist. Cross-reactivity occurs with cephalosporins in 3% to 15% of patients.

Protect from light: no

Special considerations
If concomitant aminoglycoside use is needed, administer at least 1 hour from the ampicillin sodium-sulbactam and flush tubing prior to administration.

pH: 8.0 to 10.0

Stability
Solutions made in D_5W stable for only 4 hours; stable in NS for 72 hours if refrigerated; use intramuscular and direct intravenous injection within 1 hour of reconstitution.

Solution compatibility: NS (preferred)

Compatible drugs

Aztreonam
Cefepime HCl
Enalaprilat
Famotidine
Filgrastim
Fluconazole
Fludarabine phosphate

Heparin sodium
Insulin, regular
Meperidine HCl
Morphine sulfate
Paclitaxel
Tacrolimus
Teniposide

Incompatible drugs

Amrinone lactate
Azathioprine sodium
Cefotaxime sodium
Cefoxitin sodium
Chlorpromazine HCl
Diltiazem HCl
Dobutamine HCl
Doxycycline hyclate
Ganciclovir sodium
Hydralazine HCl
Hydroxyzine HCl
Idarubicin HCl
Methylprednisolone sodium
    succinate

Midazolam HCl
Minocycline HCl
Ondansetron HCl
Pentamidine isethionate
Prochlorperazine edisylate
Promethazine HCl
Propofol
Protamine sulfate
Quinidine gluconate
Sargramostim
Verapamil HCl

AMRINONE LACTATE
Inocor®, Sanofi Winthrop Pharmaceuticals

Methods of administration
Direct intravenous injection (undiluted over 2 to 5 minutes), intermittent intravenous infusion, and continuous intravenous infusion. When amrinone is given by direct intravenous injection, administer drug undiluted over 2 to 5 minutes directly into a vein or into the tubing of a freely flowing compatible intravenous solution.

Dosing and administration
Standard: 500 mg amrinone/250 mL of NS or 0.45% NS (maximum concentration: 600 mg/200 mL of NS)

Low cardiac output states (eg, congestive heart failure)
Initiate therapy with 0.75 mg/kg as a direct intravenous injection or in 50 mL of NS administered over 15 to 20 minutes. Based on the clinical response, an additional loading dose of 0.75 mg/kg may be given 30 minutes after the initiation of therapy. Continue therapy with a maintenance infusion of 2 to 5 µg/kg/minute and slowly titrate up every 6 to 8 hours by 2.5 µg/kg/minute. Patients can usually be maintained between 10 µg/kg/minute and 15 µg/kg/minute, but should not exceed the recommended total daily dose (including loading doses) of 10 mg/kg. A limited number of patients studied at higher doses support a dosage regimen up to 18 mg/kg/day for short durations of therapy. An alternative method of administration includes administering 30 µg/kg/minute for the first 30 minutes of therapy followed by the maintenance infusion.

Onset of action occurs within minutes and peaks within 10 to 15 minutes.

Net hemodynamic effects may be synergistic with dobutamine. However, profound hypotension may occur with this combination.

Fifty percent of drug eliminated through the kidney. Administer 50% to 75% of the dose in patients with a creatinine clearance less than 10 mL/minute.

Monitor

Desired effects: increase in cardiac output and cardiac index, and decreased pulmonary wedge pressure and systemic vascular resistance.

Other monitoring parameters: blood pressure (hypotension with rapid infusions), ECG (atrial and ventricular arrhythmias), heart rate, fluid and potassium, platelet count (thrombocytopenia may occur due to decrease in platelet survival), signs of bleeding (especially with prolonged infusions; may require a decrease in dose or discontinuation of therapy if bleeding is severe), and allergic reactions (may contain sulfites).

Protect from light: yes (stable after reconstitution)

Special considerations: rate control device recommended

pH: 3.2 to 4.0

Stability

Solutions stable at room temperature for up to 24 hours after reconstitution; amrinone undergoes chemical degradation with dextrose.

Solution compatibility: NS and ½NS (*not stable* in D$_5$W)

Compatible drugs

(applies to medications in NS or ½NS diluent)

Aminophylline
Atropine sulfate
Bretylium tosylate
Calcium chloride
Cimetidine HCl
Digoxin
Dobutamine HCl
Dopamine HCl
Epinephrine HCl
Famotidine
Hydrocortisone sodium
    succinate
Isoproterenol HCl
Lidocaine HCl
Methylprednisolone sodium
    succinate
Nitroglycerin
Nitroprusside sodium
Norepinephrine bitartrate
Phenylephrine HCl
Potassium chloride
Procainamide HCl
Propranolol HCl
Verapamil HCl

Incompatible drugs

Amphotericin B
Ampicillin sodium
Ampicillin sodium-
    sulbactam sodium
Ascorbic acid
Azathioprine sodium
Aztreonam
Calcium gluconate
Cefazolin sodium
Cefmetazole sodium
Cefoperazone sodium
Cefotaxime sodium
Cefotetan disodium
Cefoxitin sodium
Ceftazidime
Ceftizoxime sodium
Ceftriaxone sodium
Cefuroxime sodium
Chlorpromazine HCl
Clindamycin phosphate
Dexamethasone sodium
    phosphate
Diphenhydramine HCl
Doxycycline hyclate
Epoetin alfa
Esmolol HCl
Folic acid
Furosemide
Ganciclovir sodium
Heparin sodium

Imipenem-cilastatin
Insulin (human)
Ketorolac tromethamine
Magnesium sulfate
Mannitol
Methicillin sodium
Metoclopramide
Metronidazole HCl
Mezlocillin sodium
Morphine sulfate
Nafcillin sodium
Ondansetron HCl
Penicillin G potassium
Penicillin G sodium
Pentamidine isethionate
Pentobarbital sodium
Phenobarbital sodium
Piperacillin sodium
Promethazine HCl
Propofol
Pyridoxine HCl
Sodium bicarbonate
Thiamine HCl
Ticarcillin disodium-
    clavulanate potassium
Ticarcillin sodium
Tobramycin sulfate
Urokinase
Vancomycin HCl

ATRACURIUM BESYLATE
Tracrium®, Glaxo Wellcome Inc.

Methods of administration

Direct intravenous injection (undiluted over 15 to 30 seconds), intermittent intravenous infusion, continuous intravenous infusion, and *not* intramuscular injection

Dosing and administration

Standard: 50 mg/250 mL of D$_5$W or NS (concentrated 100 mg/250 mL)

Immobilization for mechanical ventilation

Atracurium is an intermediate-acting, nondepolarizing, neuromuscular blocker (onset of effect: 3 to 5 minutes, duration: 25 to 35 minutes, depending on dose). Initiate at a dose of 0.4 to 0.5 mg/kg (30 to 50 mg) by direct intravenous injection. Patient can be maintained on 5 to 15 µg/kg/minute as a continuous infusion. Increase by increments of 1 to 2.5 µg/kg/minute at 1-hour intervals based on peripheral nerve stimulus using the train-of-four monitoring.

Indications for neuromuscular blocking agents in the intensive care unit include endotracheal intubation, status epilepticus, status asthmaticus, adult respiratory distress syndrome, neuromuscular toxins, tetanus, and hypothermia.

DO NOT PARALYZE PATIENT WITHOUT ADEQUATE SEDATION. Need to coadminister with medications that provide sedation, analgesia, or amnesia. Use precaution with pressure points on the eyes or skin, and provide prophylaxis for thrombosis.

Dose or interval adjustment not necessary in patients with renal or hepatic sufficiency. Clearance is independent of renal and kidney function; metabolized by both Hofmann elimination (pH [increased degradation at more alkaline pH] and temperature dependent) and ester hydrolysis.

Monitor

Neuromuscular blockade (peripheral nerve stimulation with train-of-four monitoring every 4 to 8 hours with a goal of 2 to 4 twitches), blood pressure (hypotension, secondary to histamine release and sympathetic ganglionic blockade), heart rate (tachycardia or bradycardia), manifestations of histamine release (eg, skin flushing, erythema, and pruritus), and convulsions (rare and usually in patients with predisposing factors such as head trauma).

Laudanosine is a metabolite of atracurium that is able to cross the blood-brain barrier and is elevated in patients with renal failure maintained on neuromuscular blockers for extended periods of time. Seizures and abnormal EEG response have been reported in animals with high levels of laudanosine, but are not reported in clinical trials.

Several risk factors place a patient at increased risk of prolongation of neuromuscular blockade: accumulation of drug or metabolite, electrolyte imbalance (hypokalemia, hypomagnesemia, and hypocalcemia), and medications including calcium channel blockers, corticosteroids, anti-arrhythmics (eg, procainamide and quinidine), antibiotics (eg, aminoglycosides), and immunosuppressants. Chronic use of phenytoin or carbamazepine may result in resistance to neuromuscular blockade.

Protect from light: no

Special considerations: rate control device required

pH: 3.25 to 3.65

Stability

Unstable in alkaline solutions; maximum stability at pH 2.5; stable at room temperature at concentrations of 0.5 mg/mL in compatible solutions for up to 24 hours.

Solution compatibility: D_5W, NS, D_5NS, and *not* LR

Compatible drugs

Aminophylline
Cefazolin sodium
Cefuroxime sodium
Cimetidine HCl
Dobutamine HCl
Dopamine HCl
Epinephrine HCl
Esmolol HCl
Fentanyl citrate
Gentamicin sulfate
Hydrocortisone sodium
    succinate
Isoproterenol HCl
Lorazepam
Midazolam HCl
Morphine sulfate
Nitroglycerin
Ranitidine HCl
Trimethoprim-sulfamethox-
    azole
Vancomycin HCl

Incompatible drugs

Amphotericin B
Cefoperazone sodium
Diazepam
Furosemide
Heparin sodium
Nitroprusside sodium
Pentobarbital sodium
Phenobarbital sodium
Propofol
Quinidine gluconate

ATROPINE SULFATE
various manufacturers

Methods of administration
Intramuscular (rare in ICU), subcutaneous, and direct intravenous injection

Dosing and administration
Asystole
Administer 1 mg by direct intravenous injection, and repeat every 3 to 5 minutes until rhythm returns. Intratracheal (administered in 1 mg/10 mL dilution) is 2 to 2.5 times the intravenous dose.

Bradycardia
Administer 1 mg by direct intravenous injection every 5 minutes. Repeat every 3 to 5 minutes until desired heart rate is reached, not to exceed a maximum of 3 mg or 0.04 mg/kg over 4 hours. May also give intratracheally.

Reversal of neuromuscular blockade
Administer 25 to 30 µg/kg 30 seconds before neostigmine.

Organophosphate poisoning
In moderate to severe adult overdoses, administer atropine 2 to 4 mg intravenously as a test dose. This may be doubled every 5 to 10 minutes if there is no effect until muscarinic symptoms (eg, broncheal secretions, salivation, lacrimation, urination, defecation, cramps, emesis, bradycardia, miosis) are relieved. The endpoint of therapy is reduction of bronchial secretions. Pupillary response will occur early and should not be used as a measure of adequacy of atropine dose.

In massive overdoses, hundreds of mg of atropine may be required, and it is most convenient to initiate a continuous infusion of atropine. Maximal oxygenation should be ensured prior to atropine use to minimize risk of ventricular tachydysrhythmias, (related to hypoxia). Dose tapering should be done slowly to avoid exacerbation of cholinergic symptoms.

Monitor

Heart rate (intravenous doses less than 0.5 mg and intramuscular administration of atropine have been associated with paradoxical bradycardia), orthostatic hypotension, confusion, allergic reactions (some preparations contain sodium metabisulfite), irritation at injection site, and anticholinergic syndrome, especially at higher doses (delirium, tachycardia, flushed skin, blurred vision), mydriasis and, less frequently, cycloplegia.

Protect from light: yes

Special considerations: none

pH: 3 to 6.5

Stability: incompatible with alkaline solutions; store injection at 15° to 30° C; avoid freezing

Solution compatibility

Administration with diluent as a continuous intravenous infusion is generally not recommended.

Compatible drugs

Amrinone lactate	Nafcillin sodium
Famotidine	Potassium chloride
Heparin sodium	
Hydrocortisone sodium succinate	

Incompatible drugs

Amphotericin B
Propofol

AZTREONAM
Azactam®, Bristol-Myers Squibb Company

Methods of administration
Intramuscular (dilute with ≥3 mL of diluent/g of aztreonam and inject deep into large muscle mass; pain on injection), direct intravenous injection (6 to 10 mL of sterile water for injection and infuse over 3 to 5 minutes; administer into a vein or into the tubing of freely flowing compatible intravenous solution), and intermittent intravenous infusion (administer over 20 to 60 minutes)

Dosing and administration
Standard: 1 g/50 mL and 2 g/100 mL of NS or D_5W (final concentration not to exceed 20 mg/mL)

Aztreonam is a synthetic monobactam that is active against most gram-negative aerobic bacteria, including most Enterobacteriaceae and *Pseudomonas aeruginosa*. Aztreonam is a b-lactam antibiotic and should not be considered a substitute for the aminoglycosides. Aztreonam has little or no activity against gram-positive aerobic bacteria or against anaerobic bacteria.

For treatment of the following infections: urinary tract, lower respiratory tract, skin and skin structure, intra-abdominal, and gynecological
Dosages of 500 mg to 2 g every 6 to 8 hours have been used, depending on the severity of infection. For urinary tract infections, use a dose of 500 mg to 1 g every 8 to 12 hours. For moderately severe systemic infections, use 1 to 2 g every 8 to 12 hours. For severe systemic or life-threatening infections, use 2 g every 6 to 8 hours.

May be useful in patients with allergies to penicillins and cephaloporins, as there is negligible cross-reactivity in these patients.

Dosage or interval adjustment is recommended for renal insufficiency. In patients with a creatinine clearance of 10 to 50 mL/minute, increase the interval to every 12 hours. For patients with a creatinine clearance less than 10 mL/minute, administer every 24 hours. For patients receiving hemodialysis, either give the maintenance dose after dialysis or give an additional 500 mg after dialysis if the regular dose was administered prior to dialysis. Some clinicians recommend a dose reduction of 20% to 50% in patients with hepatic failure.

Monitor
Signs of infection (temperature, white blood cell count with differential), culture and susceptibility, hypersensitivity reactions, gastrointestinal effects (nausea, vomiting, and diarrhea), and phlebitis or thrombophlebitis.

Protect from light: no

Special considerations: none

pH: 4.5 to 7.5

Stability
Reconstituted solutions are colorless to light yellow straw and may turn pink upon standing without affecting potency; lowest rate of decomposition occurs at pH of 5 to 7; stable in D_5W and NS for 24 hours at room temperature or for 7 days with refrigeration.

Solution compatibility: D_5W, NS, $D_{10}W$, D_5NS, and LR

Compatible drugs

Allopurinol sodium	Carmustine
Amikacin sulfate	Cefazolin sodium
Aminophylline	Cefepime HCl
Ampicillin sodium	Cefonicid sodium
Ampicillin sodium- sulbactam sodium	Cefoperazone sodium
	Cefotaxime sodium
Bumetanide	Cefotetan disodium
Buprenorphine HCl	Cefoxitin sodium
Butorphanol tartrate	Ceftazidime
Calcium gluconate	Ceftizoxime sodium
Carboplatin	Ceftriaxone sodium

Cefuroxime sodium
Cimetidine HCl
Ciprofloxacin
Cisplatin
Clindamycin phosphate
Cyclophosphamide
Cytarabine
Dacarbazine
Dactinomycin
Dexamethasone sodium phosphate
Diltiazem HCl
Diphenhydramine HCl
Dobutamine HCl
Dopamine HCl
Doxorubicin HCl
Doxycycline hyclate
Droperidol
Enalaprilat
Etoposide
Famotidine
Filgrastim
Fluconazole
Fludarabine phosphate
Fluorouracil
Foscarnet sodium
Furosemide
Gentamicin sulfate
Haloperidol lactate
Heparin sodium
Hydrocortisone sodium phosphate
Hydromorphone HCl
Hydroxyzine HCl
Idarubicin HCl
Ifosfamide
Imipenem-cilastatin sodium
Insulin, regular

Leucovorin calcium
Magnesium sulfate
Mannitol
Mechlorethamine HCl
Melphalan HCl
Meperidine HCl
Mesna
Methotrexate sodium
Methylprednisolone sodium succinate
Metoclopramide HCl
Mezlocillin sodium
Minocycline HCl
Morphine sulfate
Nalbuphine HCl
Ondansetron HCl
Piperacillin sodium
Piperacillin sodium-tazobactam sodium
Plicamycin
Potassium chloride
Promethazine HCl
Ranitidine HCl
Sargramostim
Sodium bicarbonate
Teniposide
Thiotepa
Ticarcillin disodium
Ticarcillin disodium-clavulanate potassium
Tobramycin sulfate
Trimethoprim-sulfamethoxazole
Vinblastine sulfate
Vincristine sulfate
Vinorelbine tartrate
Zidovudine

Incompatible drugs

Acyclovir sodium
Amphotericin B
Amrinone lactate
Amsacrine
Azathioprine sodium
Cephradine
Chlorpromazine HCl
Daunorubicin HCl
Erythromycin lactobionate
Ganciclovir sodium

Lorazepam
Metronidazole
Miconazole
Mitomycin
Nafcillin sodium
Pentamidine isethionate
Pentobarbital sodium
Prochlorperazine edisylate
Quinidine gluconate
Vancomycin HCl

BLEOMYCIN SULFATE
Blenoxane®, Bristol-Myers Squibb Company

Methods of administration
Intrapleural, intermittent intravenous infusion, intramuscular, intra-arterial, and subcutaneous

Dosing and administration
Standard: 50 mg/50 mL of NS

$$1 \text{ mg} = 1 \text{ unit}$$

Sclerosing agent for malignant pleural effusions
Prior to administration of bleomycin, confirm chest tube placement and adequate drainage of accumulated fluid. Administer an analgesic (morphine sulfate 2 to 4 mg) intravenously and 3 to 4 mg/kg lidocaine 1% intrapleurally 15 to 30 minutes prior to the procedure. Clamp the tube. Instill 50 to 60 units (not to exceed 40 units/m^2 in geriatric patients) diluted in 50 mL of NS instilled in a chest tube. Flush the tube with 10 mL NS. Clamp the tube for 6 to 12 hours. Encourage the patient to change position every 15 to 30 minutes. Reconnect the tube to water-seal drainage and suction.

Monitor
Relief of symptoms (decreased pain on respiration and improved breathing), allergic reactions, chest radiograph, pain, temperature (febrile reactions), gastrointestinal side effects (nausea, vomiting, diarrhea), alopecia, dyspnea, and drainage volume.

There is limited experience with bleomycin in effusions of nonmalignant etiology, and such use is probably less desirable than products devoid of antineoplastic actions (eg, doxycycline).

Intrapleural administration produces serum levels 30% to 40% of intravenous administration. Despite this, the medication is generally well tolerated. Myelosuppression has not been a clinical problem.

pH: 4.5 to 6 (depending on diluent)

Protect from light: no

Special preparation: none

Stability
Intact vials are stored in the refrigerator; stable for 24 hours in NS at room temperature.

Solution compatibility: NS and *not* D_5W

Compatible drugs

Not recommended to combine bleomycin with other drugs for intrapleural administration

BRETYLIUM TOSYLATE
various manufacturers

Methods of administration

Intramuscular (rotate sites), direct intravenous injection (1 to 2 minutes), intermittent intravenous infusion, and continuous intravenous infusion

Dosing and administration

Standard: 2 g in 500 mL of D_5W (4 mg/mL); maximum concentration of 2 g/250 mL

Treatment of ventricular fibrillation (typically reserved for lidocaine-refractory patients) Initiate treatment with 5 mg/kg (undiluted; typical dose of 350 to 500 mg) by direct intravenous injection over 1 minute; if arrhythmia persists after 5 minutes, give 10 mg/kg (undiluted) over 1 minute and repeat as necessary up to a maximum of 30 mg/kg. If patient responds, maintenance of 5 to 10 mg/kg (in 50 mL D_5W over 10 minutes) by intermittent intravenous infusion, every 6 to 8 hours or may be given as a continuous intravenous infusion (diluted) at a rate of 1 to 2 mg/minute. Limited experience with doses larger than 40 mg/kg/day.

Other life-threatening ventricular arrhythmias (eg, ventricular tachycardia refractory to standard therapy)
Administer 5 to 10 mg/kg in 50 mL D_5W by intermittent intravenous infusion over 8 to 10 minutes. Complete the loading dose (5 mg/kg) if bretylium appears to convert the arrhythmia and begin continuous intravenous infusion at 1 to 2 mg/minute.

May also be given intramuscularly (undiluted) at a dose of 5 mg/kg every 1 to 2 hours, with a maintenance dose of 6 to 8 hour. However, onset may require up to 2 hours.

Monitor

ECG (resolution of arrhythmia), bradycardia (most frequently seen after 30 minutes of therapy), blood pressure (supine or orthostatic hypotension, or transitory hypertension), nausea (especially with rapid intravenous infusions), lightheadedness, dizziness, vomiting, and diarrhea.

Bretylium may heighten the response to infused catecholamines and may increase the hypotensive effects of diuretics and vasodilator medications.

Rapid injection in the conscious patient may cause a decrease in blood pressure, nausea, and vomiting.

In patients with a creatinine clearance of 10 to 50 mL/minute, administer 25% to 50% of dose. In patients with a creatinine clearance less than 10 mL/minute, administer 25% of the dose. Not dialyzable (0% to 5%) via either hemodialysis or peritoneal dialysis. Supplemental doses unnecessary.

Protect from light: no

Special considerations
Use filter for ampules; rate control device recommended for continuous infusion.

pH: 4 (premixed infusion); 4.5 to 7 (injection)

Stability: generally considered to be stable over a pH range of 2 to 12

Solution compatibility: D_5W, NS, LR, and D_5NS

Compatible drugs

Amiodarone HCl	Famotidine
Amrinone lactate	Isoproterenol HCl
Diltiazem HCl	Ranitidine HCl
Dobutamine HCl	

Incompatible drugs

Amphotericin B	Promethazine HCl
Chlorpromazine HCl	Phenytoin sodium
Haloperidol lactate	Procainamide HCl
Hydroxyzine lactate	Propofol
Pentamidine isethionate	Quinidine gluconate
Prochlorperazine edisylate	

CALCIUM CHLORIDE OR CALCIUM GLUCONATE
various manufacturers

Methods of administration

Direct intravenous injection (over 5 minutes), intermittent intravenous infusion (over 20 minutes), continuous intravenous infusion (rate should not exceed 0.7 to 1.4 mEq/minute), and *not* intramuscular or subcutaneous (severe necrosis and sloughing, or leaks into the perivascular tissue)

Dosing and administration

Standard: 500 mg to 2 g/50 mL of D_5W or NS

Hypocalcemia

The dose of calcium depends on patient's clinical condition and ionized serum calcium value. For mild to moderate hypocalcemia, administer 0.5 to 1.0 g of calcium gluconate/chloride by direct intravenous injection. Repeat every 4 to 8 hours as needed. For severe, symptomatic hypocalcemia, administer 1 to 2 g calcium gluconate and repeat every hour as necessary based on symptoms and laboratory findings. As an alternative, the drug can be given by intermittent intravenous infusion or as a continuous infusion at a rate of 0.5 to 2 mg/kg/hour.

Degree of hypocalcemia based on ionized serum calcium level: mild 4.0 to 4.4 mg %, moderate 3.5 to 3.9 mg %, and severe <3.5% mg %.

Underlying causes of hypocalcemia should be identified and treated. One of the most common causes of low total serum calcium is hypoalbuminemia. If free calcium is normal, then no disorder is present. When examining total serum calcium levels in a patient with low albumin, there is a 0.8 mg/dL decrease in the calcium level for every 1 g that serum albumin concentration is less than 4 g. Other causes include renal failure and hypoparathyroidism. Hypocalcemia may also occur secondary to administration of citrate-containing blood products.

Hyperkalemia

Administer 500 mg to 1 g of calcium gluconate by direct intravenous injection. Repeat every 10 minutes as necessary based on ECG, serum potassium, and signs or symptoms of hyperkalemia.

For direct intravenous injection, do not exceed the rate of 0.7 to 1.5 mEq (approximately 50 to 100 mg of calcium chloride and 150 to 300 mg of calcium gluconate) per minute. Rapid administration may cause bradycardia.

General

Calcium gluconate and calcium chloride have different amounts of elemental calcium/mL:

1 g/10 mL (10%) calcium gluconate
9 mg calcium/mL = 0.46 mEq calcium/mL

1 g/10 mL (10%) calcium chloride
27 mg calcium/mL = 1.36 mEq calcium/mL

Prospective and retrospective studies with calcium chloride have not demonstrated benefit for cardiac arrest.

Monitor

Signs and symptoms of hypocalcemia: neuromuscular clinical manifestations (eg, paresthesias, muscle twitching, and tetany), central nervous system manifestations (eg, lethargy, seizures, confusion, agitation), and ECG changes (prolonged ST segments and QT interval).

Other monitoring parameters: blood pressure (eg, hypotension), hypomagnesemia and hyperphosphatemia (ie, confounds hypocalcemia and needs to be corrected), ionized serum calcium, serum albumin extravasation (may produce pain, necrosis, and sloughing of skin) and infusion-site irritation (calcium gluconate causes less irritation than calcium chloride).

Calcium should be used cautiously in the patient receiving digitalis because calcium increases ventricular irritability and may induce arrhythmias.

Protect from light: no

Special considerations: none

pH: calcium chloride 5.5 to 7.5
           calcium gluconate 6.0 to 8.2

Stability

Stored at room temperature for at least 24 hours; do not use if precipitate appears. Do not mix with sodium bicarbonate because precipitate will form. Do not administer in the same intravenous line as phosphate-containing solutions.

Solution compatibility: D_5W, NS, D_5NS, $D_{10}W$, and LR

Compatible drugs - calcium chloride

Amrinone lactate	Morphine sulfate
Epinephrine HCl	Paclitaxel
Esmolol HCl	

Incompatible drugs - calcium chloride

Amphotericin B	Imipenem-cilastatin sodium
Azathioprine sodium	Ketorolac tromethamine
Cefoperazone sodium	Magnesium sulfate
Ceftazidime	Methylprednisolone sodium
Ceftriaxone sodium	succinate
Cefuroxime sodium	Metronidazole
Dexamethasone sodium	Mezlocillin
phosphate	Prochlorperazine edisylate
Folic acid	Sodium bicarbonate
Haloperidol lactate	Sodium phosphate
Hydrocortisone sodium	
succinate	

Compatible drugs - calcium gluconate

Ampicillin sodium
Aztreonam
Cefazolin sodium
Cefepime HCl
Ciprofloxacin
Enalaprilat
Epinephrine HCl
Famotidine

Filgrastim
Heparin sodium
Labetalol HCl
Piperacillin sodium-
    tazobactam sodium
Potassium chloride
Sargramostim
Tacrolimus

Incompatible drugs - calcium gluconate

Amphotericin B
Amrinone lactate
Ceftriaxone sodium
Dexamethasone sodium
    phosphate
Fluconazole
Folic acid
Hydrocortisone sodium suc-
    cinate

Imipenem-cilastatin sodium
Methylprednisolone sodium
    succinate
Metoclopramide
Minocycline HCl
Prochlorperazine edisylate
Sodium bicarbonate
Sodium phosphate

CEFAZOLIN SODIUM
Ancef®, SmithKline Beecham Pharmaceuticals, and other manufacturers

Methods of administration

Intramuscular (in 2 to 5 mL sterile water and inject into large muscle mass), direct intravenous injection (in 5 to 10 mL sterile water over 3 to 5 minutes; dilute with 2 to 2.5 mL of diluent per gram of drug and infuse over 3 to 5 minutes; administer into a vein or into the tubing of freely flowing compatible intravenous solution), and intermittent intravenous infusion (over 20 to 60 minutes)

Preparation and administration

Standard: 1 g/50 mL of D_5W or NS; 2 g/100 mL of D_5W or NS

Cefazolin is a first-generation cephalosporin that has good activity against aerobic gram-positive organisms including methicillin-susceptible *Staphylococcus aureus* and *Streptococcus* sp. Cefazolin has no activity against anaerobic bacteria. Cefazolin has limited activity against gram-negative aerobic bacteria, with moderate activity against *Escherichia coli, Klebsiella* sp, *Enterobacter* sp, and *Proteus* sp.

For treatment of the following infections: urinary tract, skin and soft tissue, biliary tract, bone and joint, and endocarditis Administer 250 mg to 1.5 g every 6 to 12 hours depending on type and severity of infection. For urinary tract infections, use 1 g every 12 hours. For mild systemic infections, use 250 to 500 mg every 8 hours. For moderate to severe systemic infections, use 500 mg to 1 g every 6 to 8 hours. For life-threatening infections, use 1 to 1.5 g every 6 hours.

Perioperative prophylaxis (eg, cardiothoracic, gastric, biliary tract, vaginal and abdominal hysterectomies, cesarean section, orthopedic, craniotomy, hernia repair, and mastectomy) Administer 1 g of cefazolin by intermittent intravenous infusion 30 to 60 minutes prior to surgery. For longer surgeries, administer 1 g every 8 hours for 24 hours postoperatively.

General

Dose or frequency adjustment may be required for patients with renal insufficiency. For patients with a creatinine clearance of 10 to 30 mL/minute, increase interval to every 12 hours, and if creatinine clearance is less than 10 mL/ minute, administer every 24 hours. For patients receiving hemodialysis, either give the maintenance dose after dialysis or give an additional supplemental dose (100% of maintenance) if the regular dose is administered prior to dialysis.

Monitor

Signs of infection (temperature, white blood cell count with differential), culture and susceptibility, hypersensitivity reactions, gastrointestinal effects (nausea, vomiting, and diarrhea), and phlebitis or thrombophlebitis. Cefazolin is contraindicated for use in patients with severe, documented allergy to cephalosporin antibiotics. Cefazolin should be used cautiously in patients with allergies to penicillin or carbapenem antibiotics as cross-reactivity may exist.

Protect from light: yes (undiluted)

Special considerations

If concomitant aminoglycoside use is needed, administer at least 1 hour from the cefazolin and flush tubing prior to administration.

pH: 4.5 to 7 in sterile water, bacteriostatic water, or NS

Stability

Reconstituted solutions are light yellow in color. Solutions may darken in color without affecting potency. Stable in sterile water for injection and NS at room temperature for 24 hours, and 96 hours when refrigerated. Generally stable at pH 4.5 to 8.5.

Solution compatibility: D_5W, NS, D_5NS, $D_{10}W$, LR, $D_5^{1/2}NS$, $D_5^{1/4}NS$, and D_5LR

Compatible drugs

Acyclovir sodium
Allopurinol sodium
Amiodarone HCl (in NS)
Atracurium besylate
Aztreonam
Calcium gluconate
Cyclophosphamide
Cyclosporine
Diltiazem HCl
Enalaprilat
Esmolol HCl
Famotidine
Filgrastim
Fluconazole
Fludarabine
Foscarnet sodium
Heparin sodium

Hydromorphone HCl
Insulin, regular
Labetalol HCl
Lidocaine HCl
Magnesium sulfate
Melphalan HCl
Meperidine HCl
Morphine sulfate
Ondansetron HCl
Pancuronium bromide
Perphenazine
Sargramostim
Tacrolimus
Teniposide
Theophylline
Vecuronium bromide

Incompatible drugs

Amikacin sulfate
Amiodarone HCl (in D_5W)
Amrinone lactate
Ascorbic acid
Azathioprine sodium
Calcium chloride
Cefotaxime sodium
Cimetidine HCl
Chlorpromazine HCl
Diphenhydramine HCl
Dobutamine HCl
Dopamine HCl
Doxycycline hyclate
Erythromycin lactobionate
Ganciclovir sodium

Haloperidol lactate
Hetastarch
Hydralazine HCl
Idarubicin HCl
Minocycline HCl
Pentamidine isethionate
Pentobarbital sodium
Phentolamine mesylate
Prochlorperazine edisylate
Promethazine HCl
Protamine sulfate
Pyridoxine HCl
Quinidine gluconate
Tobramycin sulfate
Vancomycin HCl

CEFEPIME HYDROCHLORIDE
Maxipime®, Bristol-Myers Squibb Company

Methods of administration
Intramuscular (dilute with 2.5 mL D$_5$W, NS or sterile water for injection per gram of drug and inject into large muscle mass; pain on injection) and intermittent intravenous infusion (administer into a vein or into the tubing of freely flowing compatible IV solution over 20 to 60 minutes)

Dosing and administration
Standard: 1 g/50 mL or 2 g/100 mL of NS or D$_5$W (concentration should not exceed 40 mg/mL)

Cefepime is a fourth-generation cephalosporin that has excellent activity against most gram-negative aerobic organisms; including *Klebsiella* sp, *Enterobacter* sp, *Serratia* sp, *Morganella* sp, *Citrobacter* sp, and *Pseudomonas aeruginosa.* Cefepime is comparable in gram-negative activity to ceftazidime, but also has better activity against aerobic gram-positive organisms including methicillin-susceptible *Staphylococcus aureus, Streptococcus pneumoniae,* and other streptococci because of less b-lactamase induction. Cefepime is not active against anaerobic bacteria.

For the treatment of the following infections: lower respiratory tract, skin and soft-tissue, and urinary tract, including those complicated by bacteremia
Administer 500 mg to 2 g every 12 hours, depending on the severity of the infection.

For urinary tract infections, including pyelonephritis, give a dose of 500 mg to 1 g every 12 hours. For moderate to severe respiratory tract infections, dose 1 to 2 g every 12 hours; for skin and soft-tissue infections, use 2 g every 12 hours.

Dosage or interval adjustment is required for patients with renal insufficiency (creatinine clearance less than 60 mL/minute). In patients with a creatinine clearance of 30 to 60 mL/minute, administer every 12 hours. For a creatinine clearance of 11 to 29 mL/minute, change dose to 500 mg to 1 g every 24 hours. For a creatinine clearance less than 10 mL/minute, change dose to 250 mg to 500 mg every 24 hours. For patients receiving hemodialysis, dose either after dialysis or give an additional 250 to 500 mg after dialysis if the dose is given prior to dialysis. In continuous ambulatory peritoneal dialysis, the normal recommended dose should be administered every 48 hours. No dosage adjustment is required for patients with hepatic failure.

Monitor
Signs of infection (temperature, white blood cell count with differential), culture and susceptibility, hypersensitivity reactions, diarrhea, and signs of central nervous system toxicity (seizures, encephalopathy, and neuromuscular excitability).

Cefepime is contraindicated in patients with severe, documented allergy to cephalosporin antibiotics. Cefepime should be used cautiously in patients with allergies to penicillin or carbapenem antibiotics as cross-reactivity may exist.

Protect from light: yes (intact vials)

Special considerations
If concomitant aminoglycoside use is needed, administer at least 1 hour from cefepime and flush tubing prior to administration.

pH: 4.0 to 6.0 (constituted)

Stability
Reconstituted solution will range in color from colorless to amber. The color of cefepime powder and solutions may darken depending on storage conditions. However, if stored appropriately, the potency is not adversely affected. The drug is stable in D_5W, NS, $D_{10}W$, and D_5NS for 4 hours at room temperature and for 7 days if refrigerated.

Solution compatibility: NS, D_5W, $D_{10}W$, D_5NS, D_5LR, and sterile water for injection

Compatible drugs

Ampicillin sodium-sulbac-
    tam sodium
Aztreonam
Calcium gluconate
Dexamethasone sodium
    phosphate
Fluconazole
Furosemide

Hydromorphone HCl
Imipenem-cilastatin
Methylprednisolone sodium
    succinate
Piperacillin sodium-
    tazobactam sodium
Ranitidine HCl
Sodium bicarbonate

Incompatible drugs

Aminophylline
Amphotericin B
Cimetidine HCl
Ciprofloxacin
Diazepam
Diphenhydramine HCl
Dobutamine HCl
Dopamine HCl
Enalaprilat
Famotidine

Gentamicin sulfate
Haloperidol lactate
Magnesium sulfate
Meperidine HCl
Metoclopramide HCl
Metronidazole
Morphine sulfate
Ofloxacin
Tobramycin sulfate
Vancomycin HCl

CEFOTAXIME SODIUM
Claforan®, Hoechst Marion Roussel

Methods of administration
Intramuscular (diluted with 2 to 5 mL of sterile water per gram of drug and inject deep into large muscle mass; pain on injection), direct intravenous injection (10 mL of diluent and inject over 3 to 5 minutes; administer into a vein or into the tubing of freely flowing compatible intravenous solution), and intermittent intravenous infusion (20 to 60 minutes)

Dosing and administration
Standard: 1 g/50 mL of D_5W or NS; 2 g/100 mL of D_5W or NS

Cefotaxime is a third-generation cephalosporin that is active against most gram-negative aerobic organisms, including *Klebsiella* sp, *Haemophilus* sp, *Enterobacter* sp, *Serratia* sp, *Morganella* sp, and *Citrobacter* sp. Cefotaxime has poor activity against *Pseudomonas aeruginosa* and anaerobic bacteria. Cefotaxime has moderate activity against gram-positive organisms including methicillin-susceptible *Staphylococcus aureus, Streptococcus pneumoniae,* and other streptococci. Similar in spectrum of activity to ceftriaxone.

For treatment of the following infections: respiratory tract, peritonitis and other intra-abdominal, skin and skin structure, bone and joint, urinary tract, gynecological, septicemia, and central nervous system
For urinary tract and mild or uncomplicated infections, administer 1 g every 12 hours. For moderate to severe systemic infections, use 1 to 2 g every 6 to 8 hours. For severe systemic or life-threatening infections, administer 2 g every 4 to 6 hours. The duration of treatment depends on the type of infection but is usually 48 to 72 hours after resolution of infection, and the drug is typically administered for 10 to 14 days.

Gonorrhea (including strains of penicillinase-producing Neisseria gonorrhoeae*)* Administer as a single intramuscular dose of 1 g.

General

In patients with a creatinine clearance less than 20 mL/minute, reduce dose by 50%. For patients receiving hemodialysis, either give maintenance dose after dialysis or give an additional supplemental dose (50% of maintenance) if the regular dose is administered prior to dialysis. Some clinicians recommend a dose reduction of 20% to 50% for patients who have severe liver disease.

Monitor

Signs of infection (temperature, white blood cell count with differential), culture and susceptibility, hypersensitivity reactions, gastrointestinal effects (nausea, vomiting, and diarrhea), phlebitis or thrombophlebitis.

Cefotaxime is contraindicated for use in patients with severe, documented allergy to cephalosporin antibiotics. Cefotaxime should be used cautiously in patients with allergies to penicillins or carbapenem antibiotics as cross-reactivity may exist.

Protect from light: yes (excessive light only)

Special considerations

If concomitant aminoglycoside use is needed, administer at least 1 hour from the cefotaxime and flush tubing prior to administration.

pH: 5.0 to 7.5

Stability

Reconstituted solutions are light yellow to amber in color. Darkening of solutions over time may indicate a loss of potency. Do not mix with alkaline solutions or dilute in solutions with a pH greater than 7.5. Maintains potency in D_5W or NS for at least 24 hours at room temperature or for 10 days with refrigeration.

Solution compatibility: D_5W, NS, D_5NS, LR, $D_{10}W$, $D_5^{1/2}N$

Compatible drugs

Acyclovir sodium
Aztreonam
Cyclophosphamide
Cyclosporine
Diltiazem HCl
Famotidine
Fludarabine phosphate
Hydromorphone HCl
Magnesium sulfate
Melphalan HCl
Meperidine HCl
Morphine sulfate
Ondansetron HCl
Oxytocin
Perphenazine
Sargramostim
Teniposide
Tolazoline HCl
Vinorelbine tartrate

Incompatible drugs

Allopurinol
Ampicillin sodium-
    sulbactam sodium
Amrinone lactate
Azathioprine sodium
Cefazolin sodium
Ceftazidime
Ceftizoxime sodium
Chloramphenicol sodium
    succinate
Chlorpromazine HCl
Diphenhydramine HCl
Filgrastim
Fluconazole
Ganciclovir sodium
Haloperidol lactate
Hetastarch
Hydralazine HCl
Hydroxyzine HCl
Labetalol HCl
Metronidazole HCl
Methylprednisolone sodium
    succinate
Minocycline HCl
Papaverine HCl
Pentamidine isethionate
Pentazocine lactate
Pentobarbital sodium
Phenobarbital sodium
Prochlorperazine edisylate
Promethazine HCl
Protamine sulfate
Quinidine gluconate
Sodium bicarbonate
Vancomycin HCl

CEFOTETAN DISODIUM
Cefotan®, Zeneca Pharmaceuticals

Methods of administration
Intramuscular injection (dilute with 2 to 3 mL of diluent per 1 to 2 g of drug and inject deep into large muscle mass; pain occurs on injection), direct intravenous injection (10 mL of diluent per gram of drug and infuse into a vein or into the tubing of freely flowing compatible intravenous solution over 3 to 5 minutes), and intermittent intravenous infusion (over 20 to 60 minutes)

Dosing and administration
Standard: 1 g/50 mL and 2 g/100 mL of D_5W or NS

Cefotetan is a second-generation cephalosporin. Cefotetan is active against many gram-negative aerobic organisms including *Escherichia coli, Klebsiella* sp, and *Proteus* sp. Cefotetan also has moderate activity against anaerobic bacteria including *Bacteroides fragilis*, *Fusobacterium* sp, *Peptococcus* sp, *Peptostreptococcus* sp, and some *Clostridium* sp. Cefotetan also has moderate activity against streptococci and methicillin-susceptible *Staphylococcus aureus.*

For the treatment of the following infections: respiratory tract, skin and skin structure, bone and joint, urinary tract, gynecological, and intra-abdominal
Doses of 500 mg to 3 g every 12 to 24 hours have been used depending on the severity of infection. For urinary tract infections, use 500 mg to 2 g every 12 to 24 hours. For mild to moderate systemic infections, use 1 to 2 g every 12 hours. For severe systemic infections, use 2 g every 12 hours. For life-threatening systemic infections, use 3 g every 12 hours.

General
Cefotetan is relatively contraindicated for use in patients with documented allergy to cephalosporin antibiotics. Cefotetan

should be used cautiously in patients with allergies to penicillin or carbapenem antibiotics, as cross-reactivity may exist.

Dosage or interval adjustment recommended for renal insufficiency. In patients with a creatinine clearance of 10 to 50 mL/minute, administer 50% of dose. With a creatinine clearance less than 10 mL/minute, administer 25% of dose.

For patients receiving hemodialysis, administer 25% of the normal maintenance dose daily and give an additional supplemental dose (50% of maintenance dose) after each dialysis session. No adjustment necessary for hepatic failure.

Monitor
Signs and symptoms of infection (temperature, white blood cell count with differential), culture and susceptibility, hypersensitivity reactions, gastrointestinal effects (nausea, vomiting, and diarrhea), and phlebitis or thrombophlebitis. Disulfiram-type reactions have been associated with alcohol use. Hypoprothrombinemia has been associated with cefotetan disodium and other medications with the methyltetrazolethiol side chain. Hypoprothrombinemia is generally reversible with administration of vitamin K; monitor for signs of bleeding.

Protect from light: no

pH: 4.0 to 6.5 (reconstituted solutions)

Stability
Solutions may range from colorless to pale yellow. Solutions may darken in color without affecting potency. Reconstituted solutions are stable for 24 hours at room temperature or for 96 hours with refrigeration. Solutions of cefotetan in D_5W, NS, and sterile water for injection are stable for at least 1 week when frozen.

Solution compatibility: D_5W, NS, and sterile water for injection

Compatible drugs

Aztreonam
Cyclophosphamide
Diltiazem HCl
Famotidine
Fluconazole
Foscarnet sodium
Heparin sodium
Hydromorphone HCl

Insulin, human
Magnesium sulfate
Meperidine HCl
Morphine sulfate
Ondansetron HCl
Perphenazine
Teniposide

Incompatible drugs

Amphotericin B
Amrinone lactate
Azathioprine sodium
Ceftazidime (contains
    L-arginine)
Chlorpromazine HCl
Diphenhydramine HCl
Dobutamine HCl
Doxycycline hyclate
Erythromycin lactobionate
Esmolol HCl
Filgrastim
Ganciclovir sodium
Gentamicin sulfate
Haloperidol lactate
Hetastarch

Hydralazine HCl
Hydroxyzine HCl
Labetalol HCl
Minocycline HCl
Papaverine HCl
Pentamidine isethionate
Pentazocine lactate
Pentobarbital sodium
Phenobarbital sodium
Phentolamine mesylate
Prochlorperazine edisylate
Propofol
Protamine sulfate
Quinidine gluconate
Sodium bicarbonate
Tobramycin sulfate

CEFOXITIN SODIUM
Mefoxin®, Merck & Co., Inc.

Methods of administration
Intramuscular (dilute with 2 mL of sterile water per gram and inject deep into muscle mass; pain on injection), direct intravenous injection (10 mL of sterile water per gram of drug and infuse over 3 to 5 minutes; administer into a vein or into the tubing of freely flowing compatible IV solution), and intermittent intravenous infusion (over 15 to 20 minutes)

Dosing and administration
Standard: 1 to 2 g/50 mL of D_5W or NS

Cefoxitin is a second-generation cephalosporin that is active against many gram-negative aerobic organisms including *Escherichia coli, Klebsiella* sp, and *Proteus* sp. Cefoxitin also has moderate activity against anaerobic bacteria including *Bacteroides fragilis, Fusobacterium* sp, *Peptococcus* sp, and *Peptostreptococcus* sp and some *Clostridium* sp. Cefoxitin also has moderate activity against streptococci and methicillin-susceptible *Staphylococcus aureus.* Generally similar in spectrum of activity to cefuroxime and cefamandole, but more active against anaerobic pathogens.

For treatment of the following infections: respiratory tract, skin and skin structure, bone and joint, urinary tract, gynecological, septicemia, surgery prophylaxis, and intra-abdominal
Administer 1 to 2 g every 4 to 8 hours depending on the severity of infections. For urinary tract and uncomplicated systemic infections, use 1 g every 6 to 8 hours. For moderately severe or severe infections, may need to use 1 g every 4 hours or 2 g every 6 to 8 hours. Higher doses have been used for life-threatening infections (use 2 g every 4 hours or 3 g every 6 hours).

Perioperative prophylaxis (gastrointestinal surgeries, leg amputation, or abdominal and vaginal hysterectomy)
Administer 2 g 30 to 60 minutes prior to surgery, then 2 g every 6 hours for 24 hours.

Gonorrhea (including penicillinase-producing strains of Neisseria gonorrhoeae*)*
Administer a single intramuscular dose of 2 g.

General
Dose and frequency adjustment required in patients with renal insufficiency (creatinine clearance less than 50 mL/minute). In patients with a creatinine clearance of 30 to 50 mL/minute, administer 1 to 2 g every 8 to 12 hours. For a creatinine clearance of 10 to 29 mL/minute, administer 1 to 2 g every 12 to 24 hours, and if less than 10 mL/minute, give 500 mg to 1 g every 24 hours. No changes typically required in patients with hepatic failure. For patients receiving hemodialysis, either give maintenance dose after dialysis, or give an additional supplemental dose (1 to 2 g) if the regular dose is administered prior to dialysis.

Monitor
Signs of infection (temperature, white blood cell count with differential), culture and susceptibility, hypersensitivity reactions, gastrointestinal effects (nausea, vomiting, and diarrhea), and phlebitis or thrombophlebitis.

Cefoxitin is contraindicated in patients with severe, documented allergy to cephalosporin antibiotics. Cefoxitin should be used cautiously in patients with allergies to penicillin or carbapenem antibiotics as cross-reactivity may exist.

Protect from light: no

Special considerations
If concomitant aminoglycoside use is needed, administer at least 1 hour from cefoxitin and flush tubing prior to administration.

pH: 4.2 to 7.0 (reconstituted solutions); 6.5 (in premixed intravenous solution)

Stability
Solutions may range from colorless to light amber. Solutions may darken but may not necessarily affect potency or relate to

any significant chemical change. Optimal pH in range of 4 to 8. Degradation has occurred at pH less than 4 or more than 8. Reconstituted solutions are stable for 24 hours at room temperature, and for 1 week when refrigerated.

Solution compatibility: D_5W, NS, D_5NS, $D_{10}W$, $D_5^{1/2}$ NS, D_5 LR, and LR

Compatible drugs

Acyclovir sodium	Hydromorphone HCl
Aztreonam	Magnesium sulfate
Cyclophosphamide	Meperidine HCl
Diltiazem HCl	Morphine sulfate
Famotidine	Ondansetron HCl
Fluconazole	Perphenazine
Foscarnet sodium	Teniposide

Incompatible drugs

Ampicillin sodium-sulbactam sodium	Labetalol HCl
Amrinone lactate	Methylprednisolone sodium succinate
Azathioprine sodium	Minocycline HCl
Ceftizoxime sodium	Papaverine HCl
Chlorpromazine HCl	Pentamidine isethionate
Diphenhydramine HCl	Pentazocine lactate
Dobutamine HCl	Pentobarbital sodium
Doxycycline hyclate	Phenobarbital sodium
Erythromycin lactobionate	Phentolamine mesylate
Filgrastim	Prochlorperazine edisylate
Ganciclovir sodium	Propofol
Haloperidol lactate	Protamine sulfate
Hetastarch	Quinidine gluconate
Hydralazine HCl	Ranitidine HCl
Hydroxyzine HCl	Sodium bicarbonate
Insulin, human	Vancomycin HCl

CEFTAZIDIME
Fortaz®, Glaxo Wellcome Inc., and other manufacturers

Methods of administration
Intramuscular (dilute with 1.5 to 3 mL of sterile water for injection per gram of drug and inject deep into large muscle mass; pain on injection), direct intravenous injection (mix with 3 mL of diluent and inject into a vein or into the tubing of freely flowing compatible intravenous solution over 3 to 5 minutes; final concentration should not exceed 180 mg/mL), and intermittent intravenous infusion over 15 to 30 minutes

Dosing and administration
Standard: 1 g/50 mL or 2 g/100 mL of D_5W or NS (final concentration should not exceed 20 mg/mL)

Ceftazidime is a third-generation cephalosporin that has excellent activity against most gram-negative aerobic organisms, including *Klebsiella* sp, *Enterobacter* sp, *Serratia* sp, *Morganella* sp, *Citrobacter* sp, and *Pseudomonas aeruginosa*. Ceftazidime has little activity against gram-positive organisms and is not active against anaerobic bacteria.

For treatment of the following infections: serious gynecologic and intra-abdominal; severe, life-threatening infections including meningitis, hospital-acquired pneumonia, and sepsis; and infections in immunocompromised patients (neutropenic fever)
Doses of 250 mg to 2 g every 8 to 12 hours depending on the severity of infection. For urinary tract infection, use doses of 250 to 500 mg every 8 to 12 hours. For mild or uncomplicated systemic infections, use 500 mg to 1 g every 8 hours. For moderate or severe systemic infections, use 1 to 2 g every 8 to 12 hours, and for meningitis and other severe, life-threatening infections, use 2 g every 8 hours. Treatment typically continues for 10 to 14 days. Also effective in the treatment of bone and joint infections, uncomplicated pneumonia, and mild skin and skin structure infections.

Dosage or interval adjustment required for patients with renal insufficiency (creatinine clearance less than 50 mL/minute). In patients with a creatinine clearance of 31 to 50 mL/minute, reduce dose by 50% or change interval to every 12 hours. With a creatinine clearance of 16 to 30 mL/minute, reduce dose by 50% and or change interval to every 24 hours. For a creatinine clearance of 6 to 15 mL/minute, change dose to 500 mg to 1 g every 24 hours. For a creatinine clearance less than 5 mL/minute, change dose to 500 mg every 48 hours.

For patients receiving hemodialysis, either give maintenance dose after dialysis or give an additional 500 mg to 1 g after dialysis if the regular dose is administered prior to dialysis. No dosage adjustment is required in patients with hepatic failure.

Monitor
Signs of infection (temperature, white blood cell count with differential), culture and susceptibility, hypersensitivity reactions, gastrointestinal effects (nausea, vomiting, and diarrhea), and phlebitis or thrombophlebitis, and signs of toxicity (neuromuscular hyperirritability and convulsions).

Ceftazidime is contraindicated for use in patients with severe, documented allergy to cephalosporin antibiotics. Ceftazidime should be used cautiously in patients with allergies to penicillin or carbapenem antibiotics, as cross-reactivity may exist.

Protect from light: yes (intact vials)

Special considerations
If concomitant aminoglycoside use is needed, administer at least 1 hour from the ceftazidime and flush tubing prior to administration.

pH: 5 to 8 (constituted)

Stability
Solutions are light yellow to amber and may darken on storage; doesn't necessarily indicate a potency loss; stable at room

temperature in D_5W and NS for 24 hours or for 10 days when refrigerated.

Solution compatibility: D_5W, NS, and D_5NS

Compatible drugs

Acyclovir sodium	Hydromorphone HCl
Allopurinol sodium	Labetalol HCl
Aztreonam	Melphalan HCl.
Ciprofloxacin	Meperidine HCl
Diltiazem HCl	Morphine sulfate
Enalaprilat	Ondansetron HCl
Esmolol HCl	Paclitaxel
Famotidine	Ranitidine HCl
Filgrastim	Tacrolimus
Fludarabine phosphate	Teniposide
Foscarnet sodium	Vinorelbine tartrate
Heparin sodium	Zidovudine

Incompatible drugs
ceftazidime with sodium bicarbonate

Amrinone lactate	Ganciclovir sodium
Amsacrine	Haloperidol lactate
Ascorbic acid	Hydralazine HCl
Azathioprine sodium	Hydroxyzine HCl
Calcium chloride	Idarubicin HCl
Cefmetazole sodium	Midazolam HCl
Cefotaxime sodium	Minocycline HCl
Cefotetan disodium	Nitroprusside sodium
Chloramphenicol sodium succinate	Papaverine HCl
Chlorpromazine HCl	Pentamidine isethionate
Diphenhydramine HCl	Pentazocine lactate
Dobutamine HCl	Pentobarbital sodium
Doxycycline hyclate	Phenytoin sodium
Fluconazole	Prochlorperazine edisylate
	Promethazine HCl

Propofol
Protamine sulfate
Quinidine gluconate
Sargramostim

Thiamine HCl
Vancomycin HCl
Verapamil HCl

CEFTIZOXIME SODIUM
Cefizox®, Fujisawa USA, Inc.

Methods of administration
Intramuscular (dilute with 3 mL of diluent per gram of drug and inject deep into large muscle mass; pain with injection), direct intravenous injection (10 mL of diluent per gram of drug and inject into a vein or into the tubing of freely flowing compatible intravenous solution, over 3 to 5 minutes), and intermittent intravenous infusion (over 15 to 30 minutes)

Dosing and administration
Standard: 1 g/50 mL of D_5W or NS; 2 g/100 mL of either D_5W or NS

Ceftizoxime is a third-generation cephalosporin that is active against most gram-negative aerobic organisms, including *Klebsiella* sp, *Haemophilus* sp, *Enterobacter* sp, *Serratia* sp, *Morganella* sp, and *Citrobacter* sp. Ceftizoxime has poor activity against *Pseudomonas aeruginosa.* Ceftizoxime has moderate activity against gram-positive organisms including methicillin-susceptible *Staphylococcus aureus, Streptococcus pneumoniae,* and other streptococci. Ceftizoxime also has moderate activity against anaerobic bacteria including *Bacteroides fragilis*, *Peptococcus* sp, and *Peptostreptococcus* sp.

For treatment of the following infections: respiratory tract, intra-abdominal, skin and skin structure, bone and joint, and urinary tract
Dosages of 500 mg to 4 g every 8 to 12 hours depending on the severity of infection. For urinary tract infections, use 500 mg every 12 hours. For mild to moderate systemic infections, use a dose of 1 g every 8 to 12 hours. For severe systemic infections, use 1 to 2 g every 8 to 12 hours. For life-threatening infections and meningitis use 3 to 4 g every 8 hours.

Dose or frequency adjustment required in patients with renal insufficiency (creatinine clearance less than 50 mL/minute). In patients with a creatinine clearance of 10 to 50 mL/minute, administer 100% of dose every 12 hours. For a creatinine clearance less than 10 mL/minute, change interval to every 24 to 48 hours. In patients receiving hemodialysis, a supplemental dose is unnecessary if the drug is administered after hemodialysis. Otherwise, a supplemental dose (equal to the maintenance dose) can be given after dialysis. No dosage adjustment is required for hepatic insufficiency.

Monitor
Signs of infection (temperature, white blood cell count with differential), culture and susceptibility, hypersensitivity reactions, gastrointestinal effects (nausea, vomiting, and diarrhea), and phlebitis or thrombophlebitis.

Ceftizoxime is contraindicated for use in patients with severe, documented allergy to cephalosporin antibiotics. Ceftizoxime should be used cautiously in patients with allergies to penicillin or carbapenem antibiotics, as cross-reactivity may exist.

Protect from light: yes (intact vials only)

Special considerations
If concomitant aminoglycoside use is needed, administer at least 1 hour from the ceftizoxime and flush tubing prior to administration.

pH: 6 to 8

Stability
Reconstituted solutions are colorless to pale yellow in color. Solutions may turn dark yellow to amber without affecting potency. Ceftizoxime appears to be more stable at low concentrations and when reconstituted with diluents other than D_5W. Stable for 24 hours at room temperature in D_5W, $D_{10}W$, LR, and NS; stable for 96 hours with refrigeration when reconstituted in sterile water for injection.

Solution compatibility: D_5W, NS, $D_{10}W$, LR, and D_5NS

Compatible drugs

Acyclovir
Allopurinol
Aztreonam
Enalaprilat
Esmolol HCl
Famotidine
Foscarnet sodium

Hydromorphone HCl
Labetalol HCl
Meperidine HCl
Morphine sulfate
Ondansetron HCl
Sargramostim
Vinorelbine tartrate

Incompatible drugs

Amphotericin B
Amrinone lactate
Cefotaxime sodium
Cefoxitin sodium
Chlorpromazine HCl
Doxycycline hyclate
Erythromycin lactobionate
Filgrastim
Ganciclovir sodiium
Haloperidol lactate
Hydralazine HCl
Hydroxyzine HCl
Minocycline HCl
Nalbuphine HCl
Nitroprusside sodium
Norepinephrine bitartrate
Ondansetron HCl
Paclitaxel
Penicillin G potassium
Penicillin G sodium
Pentamidine isethionate
Pentazocine lactate
Pentobarbital
Phentolamine mesylate

Phenylephrine HCl
Piperacillin sodium
Piperacillin sodium-
   tazobactam sodium
Potassium chloride
Procainamide HCl
Prochlorperazine edisylate
Promethazine HCl
Propofol
Propranolol
Protamine sulfate
Pyridoxine HCl
Quinidine gluconate
Ranitidine HCl
Ritodrine HCl
Sodium bicarbonate
Succinylcholine chloride
Thiamine HCl
Tobramycin sulfate
Urokinase
Vancomycin HCl
Vasopressin
Verapamil HCl

CEFTRIAXONE SODIUM
Rocephin®, Roche Laboratories Inc.

Methods of administration

Intramuscular (dilute with 3.5 mL of diluent per gram of drug and inject deep into large muscle mass; pain on injection), direct intravenous injection (10 mL of diluent and infuse into a vein or into the tubing of freely flowing compatible intravenous solution over 4 minutes), and intermittent intravenous infusion (over 15 to 30 minutes)

Dosing and administration

Standard: 1 g/50 mL and 2 g/100 mL of D_5W or NS

Ceftriaxone is a third-generation cephalosporin that is active against most gram-negative aerobic organisms, including *Klebsiella* sp, *Haemophilus* sp, *Enterobacter* sp, *Serratia* sp, *Morganella* sp, and *Citrobacter* sp. Ceftriaxone has poor activity against *Pseudomonas aeruginosa* and anaerobic bacteria. Ceftriaxone has moderate activity against gram-positive organisms including methicillin-susceptible *Staphylococcus aureus, Streptococcus pneumoniae,* and other streptococci. Ceftriaxone has activity similar to cefotaxime.

For treatment of the following infections: bone and joint, uncomplicated gonorrhea, bacterial septicemia, peritonitis and other intra-abdominal, central nervous system, lower respiratory tract, skin and skin structure, and urinary tract
The usual adult dose is 1 to 2 g given once or twice daily depending on the type and severity of infection. Maximum of 4 g per day. For urinary tract infections and mild or moderate systemic infections, use 1 g every 24 hours. For severe systemic infections, use 2 g every 24 hours. For life-threatening infections or meningitis, 2 g every 12 hours have been used. Continue for 48 to 72 hours after patient becomes asymptomatic or evidence of eradication. Typically 10 to 14 days.

Treatment of gonorrhea (including penicillinase-producing Neisseria gonorrhoeae*)* Administer as a single intramuscular dose of ceftriaxone 125 mg to 250 mg.

General
The long half-life may facilitate long-term parenteral therapy (eg, home care).

The dose or frequency of administration of ceftriaxone, which has both renal and hepatic elimination, needs to be reduced only with both renal and hepatic insufficiency. In these patients, the daily dose should be reduced by 50%, and total daily doses should generally not exceed 2 g. Negligible removal by hemodialysis; supplemental dose is generally not required if ceftriaxone is administered after hemodialysis.

Monitor
Signs of infection (temperature, white blood cell count with differential), culture and susceptibility, hypersensitivity reactions, gastrointestinal (nausea, vomiting, and diarrhea), and phlebitis and thrombophlebitis.

Ceftriaxone is contraindicated in patients with severe, documented allergy to cephalosporin antibiotics. Ceftriaxone should be used cautiously in patients with allergies to penicillin or carbapenem antibiotics, as cross-reactivity may exist.

Biliary pseudolithiasis (presumably due to complexation of ceftriaxone with calcium-containing bile salts) may be more common in patients not eating by mouth or receiving enteral nutrition.

Protect from light: yes (intact vials); not required for reconstituted solutions

Special considerations
If concomitant aminoglycoside use is needed, administer at least 1 hour from the ceftriaxone and flush tubing prior to administration.

pH: 6.7 (1% aqueous solution); 6.6 (premixed solution)

Stability

Reconstituted solutions are light yellow to amber in color; stable in D_5W and NS for at least 24 hours at room temperature or for 3 days with refrigeration.

Solution compatibility: D_5W, NS, $D_{10}W$, D_5NS, and $D_5^{1/2}NS$

Compatible drugs

Acyclovir sodium	Methotrexate sodium
Allopurinol sodium	Morphine sulfate
Aztreonam	Paclitaxel
Diltiazem HCl	Sargramostim
Fludarabine phosphate	Sodium bicarbonate
Foscarnet sodium	Tacrolimus
Heparin sodium	Teniposide
Melphalan HCl	Vinorelbine tartrate
Meperidine HCl	Zidovudine

Incompatible drugs

Aminophylline	Ganciclovir sodium
Amrinone lactate	Haloperidol lactate
Amsacrine	Hydralazine HCl
Ascorbic acid	Hydroxyzine HCl
Azathioprine sodium	Imipenem-cilastatin sodium
Calcium chloride	Labetalol HCl
Calcium gluconate	Magnesium sulfate
Clindamycin phosphate	Metronidazole HCl
Chloramphenicol sodium succinate	Minocycline HCl
Chlorpromazine HCl	Pentamidine isethionate
Diphenhydramine HCl	Pentobarbital sodium
Dobutamine HCl	Prochlorperazine edisylate
Famotidine	Promethazine HCl
Filgrastim	Protamine sulfate
Fluconazole	Quinidine gluconate
	Tobramycin sulfate

CIMETIDINE HYDROCHLORIDE
Tagamet®, SmithKline Beecham Pharmaceuticals

Methods of administration
Intramuscular, direct intravenous injection (300 mg in 20 mL NS administered over at least 5 minutes), intermittent intravenous infusion (over 15 to 20 minutes), and continuous intravenous infusion

Dosing and administration
Standard: 300 mg/50 mL of D_5W or NS or 900 mg/100 mL to 1000 mL of D_5W or NS

Gastrointestinal disorders
Administer 300 mg every 6 to 8 hours (do not exceed 2400 mg/day). For administration by continuous infusion, administer 37.5 mg/hour (900 mg/day) and adjust to maintain an intragastric pH $\geq$5. For patients requiring a more rapid elevation of gastric pH, the continuous infusion may be preceded by a 150-mg loading dose administered by intermittent intravenous infusion.

Cimetidine has been used for prevention of stress ulceration, treatment of gastric or duodenal ulcers, and control of gastric pH in critically ill patients.

Dosage or interval adjustment is required in patients with renal insufficiency, ie, creatinine clearance less than 50 mL/minute. For patients with a creatinine clearance between 10 and 50 mL/minute, administer 50% of the dose. In patients with a creatinine clearance less than 10 mL/minute, administer 25% of the dose.

Monitor
Symptomatic response to therapy, gastric pH, signs of bleeding (eg, occult blood), central nervous system effects (eg, headache, dizziness, and confusion; mental status changes occur most frequently in elderly patients, or in patients with renal or hepatic dysfunction), hematologic effects (eg, thrombocytopenia, neutropenia), serum creatinine (monitor renal

status to correct dose), and blood pressure (eg, hypotension if administered too rapidly).

Cimetidine has the potential to impair the metabolism and increase the effects of warfarin, theophylline, lidocaine, procainamide, quinidine, phenytoin, carbamazepine, diazepam, glipizide, propranolol, and cyclosporine. Also, the increase in gastric pH will decrease absorption of ketoconazole and itraconazole but not fluconazole.

Protect from light: yes (intact vials); not required for diluted solution

Special considerations: none

pH: 3.8 to 6 (vial); 5 to 7 (premixed)

Stability
May precipitate upon exposure to cold but can be redissolved by warming without degradation. Most stable at pH of 6; stable in dilution for up to 7 days at room temperature.

Solution compatibility: D_5W, NS, $D_{10}W$, D_5LR, $D_5{}^{1/2}NS$, D_5NS, and LR

Compatible drugs

Acyclovir sodium	Fludarabine phosphate
Aminophylline	Foscarnet sodium
Amrinone lactate	Haloperidol lactate
Atracurium besylate	Heparin sodium
Aztreonam	Hetastarch
Cisplatin	Idarubicin HCl
Cyclophosphamide	Labetalol HCl
Cytarabine	Melphalan HCl
Diltiazem HCl	Methotrexate sodium
Doxorubicin HCl	Ondansetron HCl
Enalaprilat	Paclitaxel
Esmolol HCl	Pancuronium bromide
Filgrastim	Piperacillin sodium-
Fluconazole	tazobactam sodium

Compatible drugs continued

Sargramostim
Tacrolimus
Teniposide
Tolazoline
Vecuronium bromide
Vinorelbine tartrate
Zidovudine

Incompatible drugs

Amphotericin B
Amsacrine
Azathioprine sodium
Cefazolin sodium
Cefepime HCl
Cefoperazone sodium
Chlorpromazine HCl
Chloramphenicol sodium succinate
Furosemide
Ganciclovir sodium
Pentobarbital sodium
Phenobarbital sodium
Propofol

CIPROFLOXACIN
Cipro®, Bayer Corporation

Method of administration
Intermittent intravenous infusion (over 60 minutes)

Dosing and administration
Standard: 200 mg/100 mL and 400 mg/200 mL of D_5W or NS

Ciprofloxacin is a quinolone antibiotic that is active against most gram-negative aerobic bacteria, including Enterobacteriaceae and *Pseudomonas aeruginosa*. It also is active against some gram-positive aerobic bacteria, including penicillinase-producing and nonpenicillinase-producing staphylococci. Many strains of streptococci are relatively resistant to the drug. The drug is generally less active against gram-positive than gram-negative bacteria. Ciprofloxacin also has some activity against *Chlamydia* sp, *Mycoplasma* sp, *Mycobacterium* sp, *Plasmodium* sp, *Rickettsia* sp, *Salmonella* sp, and *Neisseria gonorrhoeae*.

Lower respiratory tract, skin and skin structure, bone and joint, and urinary tract infections
Administer in doses of 200 to 400 mg every 12 hours.

Administer ciprofloxacin daily in patients with a creatinine clearance less than 30 mL/minute. In patients with a creatinine clearance of 10 to 30 mL/minute, administer 100% of the dose every 12 to 24 hours. In patients with a creatinine clearance less than 10 mL/minute, administer 20% to 25% of the dose every 24 hours. Negligible removal by hemodialysis. No adjustment generally recommended in patients who have hepatic failure.

Monitor
Signs of infection (temperature, white blood cell count with differential), culture and susceptibility, gastrointestinal effects (nausea, diarrhea, abdominal pain), hypersensitivity, central nervous system effects (drowsiness, headache, and insom-

nia), and signs of central nervous system toxicity (neuro-muscular hyperirritability and convulsions).

Ciprofloxacin increases theophylline and cyclosporine serum levels and increases the effects of warfarin by interfering with hepatic metabolism.

Protect from light: yes (undiluted)

Special considerations: none

pH: For 0.2% ready-for-use infusion solution, pH is 3.5 to 4.6; for 1.0% aqueous concentrate, pH is 3.3 to 3.9.

Stability
Solutions are stable for up to 14 days after dilution at room temperature.

Solution compatibility: D_5W, NS, $D_{10}W$, and LR

Compatible drugs

Aztreonam	Potassium acetate
Calcium gluconate	Potassium chloride
Ceftazidime	Potassium phosphate
Cyclosporine	Prednisolone sodium
Digoxin	phosphate
Diltiazem HCl	Promethazine HCl
Diphenhydramine HCl	Ranitidine HCl
Dobutamine HCl	Sodium bicarbonate (D_5W)
Dopamine HCl	Sodium phosphate
Gentamicin sulfate	Tacrolimus
Hydroxyzine HCl	Teniposide
Lidocaine HCl	Tobramycin sulfate
Metoclopramide HCl	Verapamil HCl
Piperacillin sodium	

Incompatible drugs

Aminophylline
Cefepime HCl
Clindamycin phosphate
Dexamethasone sodium
    phosphate
Furosemide
Heparin sodium
Hydrocortisone sodium
    succinate
Magnesium sulfate
Methylprednisolone sodium
    succinate
Mezlocillin sodium
Phenytoin sodium
Propofol
Sodium bicarbonate (NS)

CISATRACURIUM BESYLATE
Nimbex™, Glaxo Wellcome Inc.

Methods of administration

Intermittent intravenous infusion, continuous intravenous infusion, direct intravenous injection (over 5 to 10 seconds), and *not* intramuscular injection

Dosing and administration

Standard: 50 mg/100 mL of D_5W or NS (concentrated solution 200 mg/100 mL)

Immobilization for mechanical ventilation

Cisatracurium is an intermediate-acting, nondepolarizing neuromuscular blocker (onset of effect: 2 to 3 minutes; duration: 60 minutes, depending on dose). An initial dose of 0.1 mg/kg cisatracurium with a maintenance dose of 2 to 5 µg/kg/minute typically provides adequate neuromuscular blockade in adult patients in the intensive care unit. Increase dose based on patient response as determined by peripheral nerve stimulation. Neuromuscular blockade potency is approximately three times that of atracurium.

Indications for neuromuscular blocking agents in the intensive care unit include endotracheal intubation, sedation, status epilepticus, status asthmaticus, adult respiratory distress syndrome, neuromuscular toxins, tetanus, and hypothermia.

DO NOT PARALYZE PATIENT WITHOUT ADEQUATE SEDATION. Need to coadminister with medications that provide sedation, analgesia, or amnesia. Use precaution with pressure points on the eyes or skin, and provide prophylaxis for thrombosis.

Cisatracurium causes less histamine release than atracurium and thus provides more cardiac stability. Can be administered with less volume, and is frequently less expensive.

Dose or interval adjustment not necessary in patients with renal or hepatic sufficiency. Clearance is independent of renal and liver function. Organ-dependent Hofman elimination is the predominant pathway for elimination.

Monitor

Neuromuscular blockade (peripheral nerve stimulation with train-of-four monitoring every 4 to 8 hours with a goal of 2 to 4 twitches), blood pressure (hypotension), and heart rate (tachycardia and bradycardia).

Several risk factors place a patient at increased risk of prolongation of neuromuscular blockade: accumulation of drug or metabolite, electrolyte imbalance (hypokalemia, hypomagnesemia, and hypocalcemia), and medications including calcium channel blockers, corticosteroids, anti-arrhythmics (eg, procainamide and quinidine), antibiotics (eg, aminoglycosides), and immunosuppressants. Chronic use of phenytoin or carbamazepine may result in resistance to neuromuscular blockade.

Protect from light: yes (undiluted); after dilution protection is not necessary

Special considerations: rate control device required; undiluted product requires refrigeration

pH: 3.25 to 3.65

Stability

Unstable in alkaline solutions (pH >8); may be stored in concentrations of 0.1 mg/mL at room temperature for 24 hours.

Solution compatibility: D_5W, NS, D_5NS, and *not* LR

Compatible drugs

Alfentanil HCl	Midazolam HCl
Droperidol	Sufentanil citrate

Incompatible drugs

Ketorolac tromethamine
Propofol

CLINDAMYCIN PHOSPHATE
Cleocin®, Pharmacia & Upjohn Company, and other manufacturers

Methods of administration
Intramuscular and intermittent intravenous infusion, and *not* direct intravenous injection

Dosing and administration
Standard: 300 mg to 900 mg/50 mL of D_5W or NS

Clindamycin is a semisynthetic derivative of lincomycin that is active against most aerobic gram-positive cocci, including staphylococci, *Streptococcus pneumoniae*, and other streptococci (except *Enterococcus faecalis*). The drug is also active against several anaerobic and microaerophilic gram-negative and gram-positive organisms, including *Actinomyces* sp, *Bacteroides* sp, *Fusobacterium* sp, *Propionibacterium* sp, and *Peptostreptococcus* sp. *Clostridium perfringens, Clostridium tetani, Corynebacterium diphtheriae*, and *Mycoplasma* sp are also inhibited by clindamycin.

Clindamycin has gram-positive coverage similar to erythromycin, and is active against most anaerobes, including *Bacteroides fragilis.* It is also active against methicillin-susceptible *Staphylococcus aureus* and *Staphylococcus epidermidis.*

Treatment of suspected or documented infections with aerobic gram-positive cocci and the more susceptible anaerobes
Included are diabetic foot, intra-abdominal, and skin and soft-tissue infections, aspiration pneumonia, and bacterial vaginosis. Administer 600 mg every 6 to 8 hours to a maximum of 4.8 g daily.

More severe infections, particularly those due to proven or suspected *B fragilis*, *Peptostreptococcus* sp, or *Clostridium* sp (other than *C perfringens)* may require doses as high as 900 mg every 8 hours.

General

Modification of dosage is not necessary in those patients with mild to moderate renal disease. Negligible removal by hemodialysis. Adjustment required for patients with severe liver failure; however it is not necessary for mild to moderate hepatic disease.

Monitor

Signs of infection (temperature, white blood cell count with differential), culture and susceptibility, and gastrointestinal effects (eg, diarrhea may occur in 20% to 30% of patients and resolves upon discontinuation of therapy in most circumstances; pseudomembranous colitis can occur), hypersensitivity, and thrombophlebitis. This drug is contraindicated in patients with severe, documented allergy to clindamycin.

Protect from light: no

Special considerations: none

pH: 5.5 to 7 (injection); 5.5 to 6.7 (in D_5W)

Stability

Optimal stability at pH of 4 (range 1 to 6.5); reconstituted solution stable at room temperature for 24 hours.

Solution compatibility: D_5W, NS, D_5NS, $D_{10}W$, and LR

Compatible drugs

Acyclovir sodium	Foscarnet sodium
Amiodarone HCl	Heparin sodium
Amsacrine	Hydrocortisone sodium
Aztreonam	succinate
Carbenicillin sodium	Hydromorphone HCl
Cyclophosphamide	Labetalol HCl
Diltiazem HCl	Magnesium sulfate
Enalaprilat	Melphalan HCl
Esmolol HCl	Meperidine HCl
Fludarabine phosphate	Morphine sulfate

Compatible drugs continued

Multivitamins
Ondansetron HCl
Perphenazine
Piperacillin sodium-tazobactam sodium
Sargramostim
Tacrolimus
Teniposide
Vinorelbine tartrate
Zidovudine

Incompatible drugs

Aminophylline
Amphotericin B
Amrinone lactate
Azathioprine sodium
Calcium gluconate
Ceftriaxone sodium
Chlorpromazine HCl
Ciprofloxacin
Filgrastim
Fluconazole
Ganciclovir sodium
Haloperidol lactate
Hydroxyzine HCl
Idarubicin HCl
Midazolam HCl
Minocycline HCl
Papaverine HCl
Pentamidine isethionate
Pentobarbital sodium
Phenobarbital sodium
Phentolamine mesylate
Phenytoin sodium
Prochlorperazine edisylate
Promethazine HCl
Quinidine gluconate
Tobramycin sulfate

DEXAMETHASONE SODIUM PHOSPHATE
Decadron®, Merck & Co., Inc. and other manufacturers

Methods of administration
Intramuscular, direct intravenous injection (4 mg/mL undiluted over 1 to 5 minutes), intermittent intravenous infusion (administer over 2 to 3 minutes), continuous intravenous infusion, and other routes including intra-articular, intrasynovial, intralesional, and soft-tissue injection

Dosing and administration
Standard: 4 to 10 mg/50 mL of D_5W and NS

Cerebral edema
Initiate with 10 mg dexamethasone by direct intravenous injection, intermittent intravenous infusion, or intramuscular injection, followed by 4 mg every 6 hours intravenously until adequate response. Response is usually seen within 12 to 24 hours, with dose reduction after 2 to 4 days, and discontinuation over 5 to 7 days. Best results seen if treatment is initiated within 6 hours of known increases in intracranial pressure.

Allergic conditions
Administer 4 to 8 mg dexamethasone intramuscularly on day one, then switch to oral medication when feasible. Slowly taper dose. This is typically done over approximately a 1-week period.

Dexamethasone has minimal mineralocorticoid activity. Dosage or interval adjustment generally not required in patients with renal insufficiency.

Monitor
Desired effects (eg, decreased intracranial pressure), signs of infection (may also mask signs of infection; corticosteroid may mask fever or cause leukocytosis), fluid status (may cause fluid retention), serum glucose (glucose intolerance), impaired wound healing, electrolytes (eg, hypokalemia), acid/base status (metabolic alkalosis), and central nervous system effects

(eg, psychosis, depression, euphoria).

Phenobarbital and phenytoin may reduce serum dexamethasone concentrations and may impair the therapeutic effects. Dexamethasone decreases the effects of vaccines and toxoids.

Protect from light: yes (vial)

Special considerations: none

pH: 7 to 8.5

Stability
Solution is clear and colorless; admixture stable at room temperature for at least 24 hours.

Solution compatibility: D_5W and NS

Compatible drugs

Acyclovir sodium	Morphine sulfate
Allopurinol sodium	Ondansetron HCl
Amsacrine	Paclitaxel
Aztreonam	Piperacillin sodium-tazobactam sodium
Cefepime HCl	
Cisplatin	Potassium chloride
Cyclophosphamide	Sargramostim
Cytarabine	Sodium bicarbonate
Famotidine	Tacrolimus
Filgrastim	Teniposide
Fluconazole	Vinorelbine tartrate
Fludarabine phosphate	Zidovudine
Foscarnet sodium	
Heparin sodium	
Melphalan HCl	
Meperidine HCl	
Meropenem	
Methotrexate	

Incompatible drugs

Amphotericin B
Amrinone lactate
Calcium chloride
Calcium gluconate
Cefuroxime sodium
Chlorpromazine HCl
Ciprofloxacin
Daunorubicin HCl
Diazepam
Diphenhydramine HCl
Dobutamine HCl
Doxycycline hyclate
Erythromycin lactobionate
Esmolol HCl
Gentamicin sulfate
Haloperidol lactate
Hydromorphone HCl
Hydroxyzine HCl
Idarubicin HCl
Labetalol HCl
Magnesium sulfate
Metaraminol bitartrate
Midazolam HCl
Minocycline HCl
Papaverine
Pentamidine isethionate
Pentazocine lactate
Perphenazine
Phentolamine
Prochlorperazine edisylate
Promethazine HCl
Propofol
Protamine sulfate
Quinidine gluconate
Tobramycin sulfate
Vancomycin HCl

DIAZEPAM
Valium®, Roche Products Inc. and other manufacturers

Methods of administration

Intramuscular (should be avoided unless there is no alternative; given deeply; pain on injection and slow, erratic absorption); direct intravenous injection (administer 5 mg/mL solution at 3 to 5 mg/minute, should not be injected into small veins); intermittent intravenous infusion (see stability data); and continuous intravenous infusion

Dosing and administration

Standard: 50 mg/500 mL of NS (concentrated solution: 50 mg/250 mL)

Agitation (eg, for mechanically ventilated patients on neuro-muscular blockade)
Initiate therapy at dose of 2.5 mg (mild agitation or debilitated patients) to 10 mg (moderate to severe agitation) by direct intravenous injection. Administer an additional dose of 2.5 to 5 mg every 10 minutes (maximum 10 mg) if response is inadequate. Consider other therapy (eg, haloperidol) if still inadequate response. Maintenance therapy should be based on patient response. Typically, patients require 2.5 to 5.0 mg (mild to moderate agitation) to 10 mg (severe agitation) every 3 to 6 hours.

Sedation for procedures (eg, endoscopy)
Administer 5 mg by direct intravenous injection. Repeat if inadequate response after 5 minutes to a maximum of 20 mg. The elderly, debilitated patients, or patients on concurrent narcotics should start at a lower dose (eg, 2.5 mg), and subsequent doses should be administered cautiously.

May consider infusing undiluted through a central line in patients with fluid restriction or if precipitation of the diluted solution occurs. When giving diazepam by continuous infusion, always administer a bolus dose prior to increasing the infusion rate.

Lorazepam and midazolam are generally considered the injectable benzodiazepines of choice because of the long half-life of diazepam (and long half-life of its metabolite N-desmethyldiazepam), hepatic clearance, risk of thrombophlebitis with peripheral administration, excessive sedation with scheduled dosing, and the large volume of fluid required for intravenous dilution. However, if long-term sedation is desired, diazepam may be useful. Diazepam is approximately one half the potency of midazolam.

No dosage or interval adjustment generally required in patients with renal insufficiency. Avoid in patients who have acute liver disease, and cirrhosis (if needed, give 50% of standard dose).

Monitor

Sedation, blood pressure (eg, hypotension usually secondary to rapid injection; propylene glycol, which is used as a vehicle to improve solubility of diazepam, may cause a lowering of systemic vascular resistance and decrease in blood pressure; decreases in blood pressure may also be seen in patients with a hypovolemic, hypothermic, or vasoconstricted state), tolerance (develops in response to the nonanxiolytic actions, not generally because of the anxiolytic actions), respiratory depression (usually occurs at high doses or with concomitant central nervous system depressants such as narcotics), pulmonary and cardiovascular compromise, and paradoxical central nervous system excitation, agitation or delirium (especially in the elderly).

pH: 6.2 to 6.9

Protect from light: yes (undiluted)

Special considerations

Use glass or polyolefin containers; avoid intra-arterial administration of benzodiazepines because it may produce spasm with resultant gangrene that may require intervention.

Stability

Most stable at pH 4 to 8. Hydrolysis occurs at pH <3. Dilution causes concentration-dependent precipitation. Mix diazepam by adding diluent to the diazepam injection; adding diazepam to diluent results in a yellow precipitate; use immediately upon mixing.

Solution compatibility: NS (if dilution is necessary)

Compatible drugs

Dobutamine HCl
Nafcillin sodium
Quinidine gluconate

Incompatible drugs

Atracurium besylate
Benzquinamide HCl
Buprenorphine HCl
Cefepime HCl
Dexamethasone sodium
  phosphate
Diltiazem HCl
Doxapram HCl
Doxorubicin HCl
Epinephrine
Esmolol HCl
Fluconazole
Fluorouracil
Foscarnet sodium
Furosemide

Glycopyrrolate
Heparin sodium
Hydromorphone HCl
Ketorolac tromethamine
Meperidine HCl
Meropenem
Metaraminol
Nalbuphine HCl
Oxytocin
Pancuronium bromide
Potassium chloride
Propofol
Ranitidine HCl
Thiamine
Vercuronium bromide

DIGOXIN
Lanoxin®, Glaxo Wellcome Inc., and other manufacturers

Methods of administration
Direct intravenous injection, intermittent intravenous infusion, and intramuscular (may cause intense pain and fasciculations; use only if other routes are not an option)

Dosing and administration
Standard: 250 µg/10 mL

Atrial fibrillation and flutter, and as an inotrope in congestive heart failure
Digitalization should occur over a 12- to 24-hour period in patients with no measurable serum drug concentrations. For patients with a creatinine clearance less than 10 mL/minute, initiate with 7.5 to 10 µg/kg lean body weight.

Patients with good renal function can start at 10 to 15 µg/kg lean body weight in divided doses. Fifty percent of the total dose can be given initially, followed by 50% of the remainder administered in 6- to 8-hour intervals. This allows for complete tissue distribution and observation of clinical effects of the preceding dose. The maintenance dose depends on renal status and serum drug concentrations, and is typically 0.125 to 0.25 mg daily.

Hypokalemia and hypomagnesemia will increase the likelihood of digoxin toxicity and should be corrected prior to initiation of therapy. Digoxin toxicity may result in gastrointestinal disturbances (eg, diarrhea and vomiting), which may also decrease the serum potassium level.

Digoxin can be given by direct intravenous injection at a rate not exceeding 1 mL/ minute (over at least 5 minutes) or preferably combined with 10 mL of NS and administered by slow intermittent infusion. Rapid administration may result in myocardial depression (secondary to 40% propylene glycol found in commercial products).

Monitor

Desired effects: atrial fibrillation and flutter — ECG and cardiac monitor. Congestive heart failure: signs of pulmonary congestion, diuresis (urinary output and weight loss), and decrease in the symptoms of dyspnea and orthopnea.

Other monitoring parameters: ECG (dysrhythmias, including AV block), heart rate (bradycardia may indicate toxicity), gastrointestinal effects (anorexia, nausea, and vomiting), electrolytes (potassium, magnesium, and calcium), central nervous system (confusion), and serum digoxin concentration.

Concomitant digoxin and quinidine therapy may increase serum digoxin levels up to twofold; maintenance doses of digoxin may need to be reduced by 50%. Serum digoxin levels may increase as much as 20% over 48 hours when diltiazem is added to the regimen. If verapamil is added to the regimen, there may be an increase of 50%. Other medications known to increase digoxin serum concentrations include amiodarone, captopril, and propafenone.

Therapeutic drug monitoring considerations
> Sample collection:
>> Trough within 60 minutes prior to dose (at least 8 hours after previous dose)
>
> Therapeutic range:
>> Congestive heart failure: 0.8 to 1.5 ng/mL
>> Arrhythmias: 1.5 to 2.5 ng/mL

Protect from light: yes (ampules)

Special considerations: none

pH: 6.8 to 7.2

Stability
Not stable in acidic solutions (pH <3); dilution to a more than fourfold volume of diluent may lead to precipitation of digoxin.

Solution compatibility: D_5W, NS, $D_{10}W$, LR, and $^1/_2$NS

Compatible drugs

Amrinone lactate
Ciprofloxacin
Diltiazem HCl
Famotidine
Heparin sodium
Insulin, regular

Meperidine HCl
Meropenem
Milrinone
Morphine sulfate
Potassium chloride
Tacrolimum

Incompatible drugs

Amphotericin B
Dobutamine HCl
Fluconazole
Foscarnet sodium

Minocycline HCl
Pentamidine isethionate
Propofol

DIGOXIN IMMUNE FAB
Digibind®, Glaxo Wellcome Inc.

Method of administration
Intermittent intravenous infusion (over 15 to 30 minutes)

Dosing and administration
Standard: 10 mg/10 mL

Acute treatment of life-threatening digitalis toxicity
Each vial (40 mg) of digoxin immune fab will bind with approximately 0.6 mg of digoxin. Digoxin immune fab dose is determined by estimating the amount of digitalis glycoside in the body, either through calculating total body load of glycoside with known serum drug concentration (Equation A) or through an estimated amount of drug ingested (Equation B).

Equation A: *Serum digoxin concentration known*

Number of Digibind® vials =

$$\frac{\text{digoxin serum concentration (ng/mL)} \times \text{TBW (kg)}}{100}$$

If digitoxin is ingested, divide numerator by 1000 instead of 100; TBW = total body weight

Equation B: *Estimated amount of digoxin ingested*

$$\text{Number of Digibind® vials} = \frac{\text{amount ingested (mg)} \times F}{0.6}$$

F = 0.8 digoxin tablets
F = 1 for digoxin elixir and capsules
F = 1 for digitoxin

If serum drug concentration and amount ingested are unknown, an empiric dose of 10 vials may be administered, followed by another 10 vials if no response is identified.

Improvement in signs and symptoms occurs within 30 minutes of antibody administration with complete reversal at 4 hours. Additional doses (25% to 50% of original) should be considered if patient does not respond adequately or if symptoms reappear within 4 hours.

Monitor

EKG (eg, AV block, PVCs), factors that increase myocardial sensitivity (hypokalemia, hypomagnesemia), and hypersensitivity or other allergic reactions (especially in patients with known allergy to sheep or in patients who have previously received digoxin immune fab).

Congestive heart failure or atrial fibrillation may be precipitated by removal of the pharmacological effects of digitalis glycosides.

Serum potassium concentrations may decrease within the first 24 hours after administration secondary to potassium shifts back into cells. This requires careful monitoring for the first several hours after administration and possible supplementation. If hypokalemia is treated, it should be done cautiously since hyperkalemia can develop rapidly in advanced digitalis toxicity.

After administration of digoxin immune fab, total serum digoxin levels are no longer meaningful since they represent both free and bound digoxin. Free (unbound) digoxin can be measured when serum level monitoring is required.

Although initial free digoxin concentrations are near zero, they begin to reappear within 5 to 24 hours or longer after digoxin immune fab administration, depending on antibody dose, infusion technique, and the patient's renal function. In patients with renal insufficiency, free digoxin concentrations will gradually rise and may not peak for 7 days. Distribution pharmacokinetics may be altered.

Protect from light: no

Special considerations: administer through 0.22 micron filter

pH: 6.8 to 7.2

Stability

The 40-mg vial of digoxin immune fab should be reconstituted in sterile water for injection and must either be immediately used or, if refrigerated, used within 4 hours of being reconstituted. This preparation can be further diluted with NS to a convenient volume (eg, 1 mg/mL).

Solution compatibility: sterile water

Drug compatibility

Limited data available

DILTIAZEM HYDROCHLORIDE
Cardizem®, Hoechst Marion Roussel

Methods of administration
Direct intravenous injection (over 2 to 5 minutes) and continuous intravenous infusion

Dosing and administration
Standard: 100 mg/250 mL of D_5W or NS (maximum concentration: 125 mg/125 mL)

Supraventricular tachycardia (SVT) and to control ventricular rate in atrial fibrillation/atrial flutter
Administer 0.25 mg/kg actual body weight by direct intravenous injection over 2 minutes (20 mg is a typical dose). If response is inadequate, a second intravenous dose of 0.35 mg/kg may be administered after 15 minutes (25 mg for the average patient).

Maintenance therapy should be started immediately after the load in patients with atrial fibrillation or flutter to maintain a controlled rate. The recommended initial infusion rate of diltiazem is 10 mg/hour. Some patients may respond to 5 mg/hour. The infusion rate may be increased in increments of 5 mg/hour up to 15 mg/hour as needed, if further reduction in heart rate is required. Maintenance doses larger than 15 mg/hour and a duration longer than 24 hours are associated with increased risk for accumulation of metabolites and increased toxicity.

Response to therapy occurs in approximately 5 minutes. Effects will be additive with digoxin and β–blockers. Use cautiously in patients with ventricular dysfunction, severe hypotension, second- or third-degree AV block, bradycardia, or heart failure.

Monitor
ECG (bradycardia, AV block), blood pressure (risk of hypotension; check every 5 to 10 minutes for 20 to 30 minutes after medication administration), factors contributing to new onset

SVT (ie, acid-base disturbances, sepsis), generalized fatigue, and headache.

Protect from light: no

Special considerations: rate control device recommended

pH: 3.7 to 4.1

Stability
Intact vials should be refrigerated; physically compatible for 24 hours at room temperature with compatible diluents; manufacturer recommends refrigeration and use within 24 hours.

Solution compatibility: D_5W, NS, and $D_5^{1/2}NS$

Compatible drugs

Acylovir (diltiazem ≤ 1 mg/mL)	Doxycycline hyclate
Albumin	Epinephrine HCl
Amikacin sulfate	Erythromycin lactobionate
Amphotericin B	Esmolol HCl
Aztreonam	Fluconazole
Bretylium tosylate	Gentamicin sulfate
Bumetanide	Hetastarch
Cefazolin sodium	Imipenem-cilastatin sodium
Cefotaxime sodium	Lidocaine HCl
Cefotetan disodium	Lorazepam
Cefoxitin sodium	Meperidine HCl
Ceftazidime	Metoclopramide HCl
Ceftriaxone sodium	Metronidazole
Cefuroxime sodium	Mezlocillin sodium
Cimetidine HCl	Morphine sulfate
Ciprofloxacin	Nitroglycerin
Clindamycin phosphate	Nitroprusside sodium
Digoxin	Norepinephrine bitartrate
Dobutamine HCl	Oxacillin sodium
Dopamine HCl	Penicillin G potassium
	Pentamidine isethionate

Piperacillin sodium
Potassium chloride
Potassium phosphate
Procainamide HCl
Ranitidine HCl
Ticarcillin disodium

Ticarcillin disodium-
    clavulanate potassium
Tobramycin sulfate
Trimethoprim-sulfamethox-
    azole
Vancomycin HCl

Incompatible drugs

Acetazolamide sodium
Acyclovir sodium (diltiazem
    > 1 mg/mL)
Aminophylline
Ampicillin sodium
Ampicillin sodium-
    sulbactam sodium
Cefamandole nafate
Cefoperazone sodium
Diazepam
Furosemide

Heparin sodium
Hydrocortisone sodium
    succinate
Insulin, regular (NS)
Methylprednisolone
    sodium succinate
Nafcillin sodium
Phenytoin sodium
Rifampin
Sodium bicarbonate
Thiopental

DIPHENHYDRAMINE HYDROCHLORIDE
Benadryl®, Parke-Davis, and other manufacturers

Methods of administration
Intramuscular (deep), direct intravenous injection (50 mg over 30 seconds, larger doses over 1 to 5 minutes), intermittent intravenous infusion, continuous intravenous infusion, and *not* subcutaneous (irritation)

Dosing and administration
Standard: 50 mg/50 mL of D_5W or NS

Allergic reactions, anaphylaxis, premedication prior to amphotericin B, acute dystonic reactions, and pruritus
Administer 25 to 50 mg intravenously. Repeat in 30 to 60 minutes if inadequate response. Administer every 6 hours as needed. For treatment of anaphylaxis, diphenhydramine is used concomitantly with epinephrine and corticosteroids.

Sedation
Administer 25 to 50 mg intravenously over 30 seconds and repeat in 30 minutes if inadequate response.

Maximum adult dose is 400 mg daily. Dosage and interval adjustment generally not required in patients with renal insufficiency.

Monitor
Desired response (eg, sedation, or reduction of clinical manifestations of an allergic condition), blood pressure (hypotension, especially in elderly with intravascular volume depletion), increase in thickness of respiratory secretions (use caution in patients with asthma), and allergic reactions (some preparations contain bisulfites).

Protect from light: yes

Special considerations: none

pH: 5 to 6

Stability: admixture stable for at least 24 hours at room temperature

Solution compatibility: D_5W, NS, $D_{10}W$, LR, and $^1/_2$NS

Compatible drugs

Acyclovir sodium
Amsacrine
Ceftazidime
Cisplatin
Cyclophosphamide
Ciprofloxacin
Cytarabine
Doxorubicin HCl
Filgrastim
Fluconazole
Fludarabine phosphate
Heparin sodium
Hydrocortisone sodium
    succinate
Hydroxyzine
Idarubicin HCl
Meperidine HCl
Melphalan HCl
Meropenem
Methotrexate
Ondansetron HCl
Paclitaxel
Piperacillin sodium-
    tazobactam sodium
Potassium chloride
Sargramostim
Tacrolimus
Teniposide
Vinorelbine tartrate

Incompatible drugs

Ampicillin sodium
Amrinone lactate
Azathioprine sodium
Aminophylline
Amphotericin B
Aztreonam
Cefazolin sodium
Cefepime HCl
Cefmetazole sodium
Cefoperazone sodium
Cefotaxime sodium
Cefotetan disodium
Cefoxitin sodium
Ceftriaxone
Cefuroxime sodium
Chloramphenicol
Dexamethasone sodium
    phosphate
Diazepam
Furosemide
Ganciclovir sodium
Haloperidol
Insulin, human
Ketorolac tromethamine
Methylprednisolone sodium
    succinate
Metronidazole HCl
Mezlocillin sodium

Nitroprusside sodium
Pentobarbital sodium
Phenobarbital sodium
Phenytoin sodium
Prochlorperazine

Promazine
Promethazine
Propofol
Sodium bicarbonate
Thiopental sodium

DOBUTAMINE HYDROCHLORIDE
Dobutrex®, Eli Lilly and Company, and
other manufacturers

Method of administration
Continuous intravenous infusion

Dosing and administration
Standard: 500 mg/250 mL (concentrated solution: 1250 mg/250 mL)

Congestive heart failure, cardiogenic shock, cardiomyopathy, or other low cardiac output states
Typically administered at 5 µg/kg/minute and titrated to response by increments of 2.5 µg/kg/minute at 10-minute intervals (maximum of 20 µg/kg/minute, rare cases of 40 µg/kg/minute).

The continuous intravenous infusion should be tapered slowly, by a rate of 2 µg/kg/minute every 20 to 30 minutes while assessing mean arterial pressure, heart rate, pulmonary capillary wedge pressure, and cardiac index to make sure that the patient remains hemodynamically stable.

Dobutamine-induced inotropic effects and increase in heart rate may increase oxygen demand in patients with a history of coronary artery disease, which may precipitate myocardial ischemia, and cardiac dysrhythmias.

Monitor
Desired effect (increase in cardiac output and stroke volume, and reductions in pulmonary capillary wedge pressure and systemic vascular resistance), heart rate (typical increase of 5 to 15 beats per minute), blood pressure (variable effect), ECG (arrhythmias), nausea, vomiting, tingling sensation, dyspnea, and allergic reaction (may contain sulfites).

Dobutamine may potentiate hypokalemia. Tolerance to hemodynamic effects may occur with long-term (72 to 96 hours) use, and is likely to be due to down regulation of β_1 receptors.

Protect from light: no

Special considerations: rate control device recommended

pH: 2.5 to 5.5

Stability
Pink color does not affect drug potency; not stable in alkaline solutions; reconstituted solutions should be used within 24 hours after preparation.

Solution compatibility: D_5W, NS, LR, $D_5{}^{1/2}$ NS, D_5NS, and $D_{10}W$

Compatible drugs

Amiodarone HCl	Labetalol HCl
Amrinone lactate	Lidocaine HCl
Atracurium besylate	Magnesium sulfate
Aztreonam	Meperidine HCl
Bretylium tosylate	Meropenem
Calcium chloride	Nitroglycerin
Calcium gluconate	Nitroprusside sodium
Ciprofloxacin	Pancuronium bromide
Diazepam	Potassium chloride
Diltiazem HCl	Ranitidine HCl
Dopamine HCl	Streptokinase
Enalaprilat	Tacrolimus
Famotidine	Vecuronium bromide
Fluconazole	Verapamil HCl
Haloperidol lactate	Zidovudine
Insulin, regular	

Incompatible drugs

Acyclovir sodium
Alteplase
Aminophylline
Amphotericin B
Ampicillin sodium
Ampicillin sodium-
    sulbactam sodium
Azathioprine sodium
Bumetanide
Cefamandole nafate
Cefazolin sodium
Cefepime HCl
Cefmetazole sodium
Cefoperazone sodium
Cefotetan disodium
Cefoxitin sodium
Ceftazidime
Ceftriaxone sodium
Cefuroxime
Chloramphenicol sodium
    succinate
Dexamethasone sodium
    phosphate
Digoxin
Folic acid
Foscarnet sodium

Furosemide
Ganciclovir sodium
Heparin sodium
Hydrocortisone sodium suc-
    cinate
Imipenem-cilastatin sodium
Ketorolac tromethamine
Methicillin sodium
Mezlocillin
Nafcillin sodium
Penicillin G potassium
Penicillin G sodium
Pentobarbital sodium
Phenobarbital sodium
Phenytoin sodium
Phytonadione
Piperacillin sodium
Piperacillin sodium-
    tazobactam sodium
Potassium phosphate
Propofol
Sodium bicarbonate
Ticarcillin disodium
Ticarcillin disodium-
    clavulanate potassium

DOPAMINE HYDROCHLORIDE
Intropin®, Faulding Pharmaceutical Co, and other manufacturers

Method of administration
Continuous intravenous infusion

Dosing and administration
Standard: 400 mg/250 mL of D_5W
(concentrated solution: 1600 mg/250 mL of D_5W)

Treatment of sepsis or cardiogenic shock, for renal insufficiency, or as an inotropic agent
The dose depends on desired effects (vasoactive, chronotropic, or inotropic effects).

To increase urine output (predominance of dopaminergic effects), use low doses of 0.5 to 3 µg/kg/minute. Stimulates receptors primarily in the renal, splanchnic, and coronary vascular beds to produce vasodilation, improved blood flow, and natriuresis. This dose may slightly increase contractility, but will have negligible effects on heart rate and systemic vascular resistance.

To increase cardiac output (predominance of β-1 and dopaminergic effects), use moderate doses of 3 to 10 µg/kg/minute. Will increase stroke volume and heart rate.

For vasoconstriction resulting in increased blood pressure (via α-1 stimulation), use a high dose of 5 to 10 µg/kg/minute or greater. Titrate at increments of 2.5 to 10 µg/kg/minute every 5 to 15 minutes (maximum 40 µg/kg/minute). Urine output is diminished by renal vasoconstriction.

The range of receptor activity overlaps the dosing ranges. Dosing should be titrated to the minimum effective dose without producing undesirable effects.

To avoid acute hypotension, taper dopamine gradually.

Monitor

Blood pressure, cardiac output (increased at moderate doses, may diminish at high doses), urine output (increased at low doses, decreased at high doses), heart rate (increased at moderate to high doses, tachycardia, and myocardial ischemia [see next paragraph]), blood pressure (increased at moderate and high doses), ECG (dysrhythmias), allergic reaction (some products contain sulfites), nausea and vomiting, ischemia of extremities with prolonged infusions. Tissue necrosis and sloughing with interstitial extravasation.

Patients with pre-existing or underlying myocardial ischemia or dysrhythmias may be particularly susceptible to adverse effects. Pulmonary edema may worsen if dopamine is administered in this setting as the drug may increase pulmonary capillary wedge pressure. Also, oxygenation (pO_2) may worsen.

Protect from light: yes

Special considerations

Infuse through a central line if possible; rate control device recommended.

pH: 2.5 to 4.5 (vials); 3 to 5 (premixed)

Stability

Dark yellow solutions indicate degradation; incompatible with alkaline solutions (may be indicated by pink discoloration); stable over a pH range of 4 to 6.4; optimal stability at pH of 5 or below.

Solution compatibility: D_5W, NS, LR, $D_5^{1/2}NS$, and $D_{10}W$

Compatible drugs

Amiodarone HCl
Amrinone lactate
Atracurium besylate
Aztreonam
Ciprofloxacin
Diltiazem HCl
Dobutamine HCl
Enalaprilat
Esmolol HCl
Famotidine
Fluconazole
Foscarnet sodium
Haloperidol lactate
Heparin sodium
Hydrocortisone sodium
  succinate
Labetalol HCl
Lidocaine HCl
Meperidine HCl
Meropenem
Midazolam HCl
Morphine sulfate
Nitroglycerin
Nitroprusside sodium
Norepinephrine bitartrate
Pancuronium bromide
Piperacillin sodium-
  tazobactam sodium
Potassium chloride
Ranitidine HCl
Sargramostim
Streptokinase
Tacrolimus
Vecuronium bromide
Verapamil HCl
Zidovudine

Incompatible drugs

Acyclovir sodium
Alteplase
Amphotericin B
Ampicillin sodium
Azathioprine sodium
Cefazolin sodium
Cefepime HCl
Cefoperazone sodium
Chloramphenicol sodium
  succinate
Ganciclovir sodium
Gentamicin sulfate
Penicillin G potassium
Propofol
Sodium bicarbonate

DOXACURIUM CHLORIDE
Nuromax®, Glaxo Wellcome

Method of administration
Direct intravenous injection (over 5 to 10 seconds)

Dosing and administration
Standard: 1 mg/mL

Immobilization for mechanical ventilation

Doxacurium is a long-acting nondepolarizing neuromuscular blocker (onset of effect: 5 to 11 minutes; duration: 120 to 150 minutes, depending on dose). Initiate blockade with a dose of 0.05 mg/kg by intravenous injection. A typical maintenance dose is 0.005 to 0.01 mg/kg as necessary. The first maintenance dose is usually needed 60 to 120 minutes after the initial dose.

Indications for neuromuscular blocking agents in the intensive care unit include endotracheal intubation, status epilepticus, status asthmaticus, adult respiratory distress syndrome, neuromuscular toxins, tetanus, and hypothermia. Typically not used because of the long duration of activity. Because of the long half-life, would only be used in patients in which extended neuromuscular blockade is anticipated..

DO NOT PARALYZE PATIENT WITHOUT ADEQUATE SEDATION. Need to coadminister with medications that provide sedation, analgesia, or amnesia. Use precaution with pressure points on the eyes or skin, and provide prophylaxis for thrombosis.

Dosage should be reduced 50% in patients with renal (creatinine clearance <50 mL/minute) or hepatic insufficiency and in the elderly.

Monitor
Neuromuscular blockade (peripheral nerve stimulation with train-of-four monitoring every 4 to 8 hours with a goal of 2 to 4 twitches), blood pressure (hypotension), and heart rate (tachycardia and bradycardia).

Several risk factors place a patient at increased risk of prolongation of neuromuscular blockade: accumulation of drug or metabolite, electrolyte imbalance (hypokalemia, hypomagnesemia, and hypocalcemia), and medications including calcium channel blockers, corticosteroids, antiarrhythmics (eg, procainamide and quinidine), antibiotics (eg, aminoglycosides), and immunosuppressants. Chronic use of phenytoin or carbamazepine may result in resistance to neuromuscular blockade.

Minimal histamine-release hypotension or vagal-block tachycardia. Advantage in patients considered to be cardiovascularly compromised.

Protect from light: no

Special considerations: none

pH: 3.9 to 5.0 (in sterile water for injection)

Stability
May not be compatible with alkaline solutions with a pH >8.5.

Solution compatibility: D$_5$W, NS, D$_5$NS, and LR

Compatible drugs

Etomidate
Thiopental sodium

Incompatible drugs

Limited data available

DOXYCYCLINE HYCLATE
Vibramycin®, Pfizer Inc, and other manufacturers

Methods of administration
Intrapleural and intermittent intravenous infusion (over 60 minutes)

Dosing and administration
Standard: 100 mg/250 mL of D_5W or NS

Doxycycline is a semisynthetic tetracycline that is active against most *Mycoplasma* sp, *Chlamydia* sp, *Rickettsia* sp, spirochetes, and many gram-positive bacteria. Doxycycline (or erythromycin) is the treatment of choice for *Mycoplasma pneumoniae* and *Chlamydia trachomatis.* Doxycycline is an alternative choice for *Streptococcus pneumoniae* (note that penicillin-resistant strains may also be resistant to doxycycline) and *Legionella* sp (erythromycin is treatment of choice).

Treatment of bronchitis, pelvic inflammatory disease, and urethritis caused by susceptible organisms
The usual dosage of intravenous doxycycline is 200 mg on the first day of treatment administered in one or two intermittent infusions over 1 hour. Subsequent daily dosage is 100 to 200 mg, depending upon the severity of infection, with 200 mg administered in one or two infusions.

Sclerosing agent for treatment of malignant or nonmalignant pleural effusions
Prior to administration of doxycycline, confirm chest tube placement and adequate drainage of accumulated fluid. Administer an analgesic (morphine sulfate 2 to 4 mg intravenously) and 3 to 4 mg/kg lidocaine 1% intrapleurally 15 to 30 minutes prior to the procedure. Clamp the tube. Instill 500 mg to 1 g doxycycline with 25 to 30 mL of NS. Flush the tube with 10 mL NS. Clamp the tube for 6 to 12 hours. Encourage the patient to change position every 15 to 30 minutes. Reconnect the tube to water-seal drainage and suction.

General

No dosage adjustment is necessary in patients with renal insufficiency. Negligible removal by hemodialysis (0% to 5%).

Doxycycline can cause fetal toxicity when administered to pregnant women.

Monitor

For intrapleural administration: relief of symptoms, allergic reactions, pain, fever, and drainage volume. For treatment of infection: signs and symptoms (eg, temperature, white blood cell count with differential), culture and susceptibility, hypersensitivity reactions, and gastrointestinal effects.

Doxycycline is contraindicated for use in patients with severe, documented allergy to the tetracycline antibiotics. Pregnancy category D.

Protect from light: yes (protect from direct sunlight)

Special considerations: none

pH: 1.8 to 3.3 (reconstituted with sterile water)

Stability

Stable at room temperature for 48 hours when mixed with compatible diluents.

Solution compatibility: D_5W, NS, and D_5NS

Compatible drugs

Acyclovir sodium	Melphalan HCl
Amiodarone HCl	Meperidine HCl
Aztreonam	Morphine sulfate
Cyclophosphamide	Ondansetron HCl
Diltiazem HCl	Perphenazine
Filgrastim	Sargramostim
Fludarabine phosphate	Tacrolimus
Hetastarch	Teniposide
Hydromorphone HCl	Vinorelbine tartrate
Magnesium sulfate	

Incompatible drugs

Amphotericin B
Ampicillin sodium
Ampicillin sodium-
    sulbactam sodium
Amrinone lactate
Azathioprine sodium
Cefazolin sodium
Cefmetazole sodium
Cefoperazone sodium
Cefotetan disodium
Cefoxitin sodium
Ceftazidime
Ceftizoxime sodium
Cefuroxime sodium
Chloramphenicol sodium
    succinate
Dexamethasone sodium
    phosphate
Erythromycin lactobionate
Folic acid
Furosemide
Ganciclovir sodium
Heparin sodium
Hydrocortisone sodium
    succinate
Ketorolac tromethamine
Methicillin sodium
Methylprednisolone sodium
    succinate
Mezlocillin sodium
Moxalactam disodium
Nafcillin sodium
Oxacillin sodium
Penicillin G potassium
Penicillin G sodium
Pentobarbital sodium
Phenobarbital
Piperacillin sodium
Piperacillin sodium-
    tazobactam sodium
Sodium bicarbonate

ENALAPRILAT
Vasotec®, Merck & Co., Inc.

Methods of administration
Direct intravenous injection (over at least 5 minutes if undiluted) and intermittent intravenous infusion.

Dosing and administration
Standard: Dose/50 mL of D_5W or NS

Mild to moderate hypertension and afterload reduction in left ventricular dysfunction
Initiate at 1.25 mg by direct intravenous injection over 5 minutes or intermittent intravenous infusion over 15 to 30 minutes every 6 hours. Patients with concomitant diuretic therapy or who have clinical evidence of hypovolemia should start therapy at 0.625 mg. Concomitant diuretic therapy may enhance response. Dose can be titrated by increments of 1.25 mg at 12- to 24-hour intervals for a maximum dose of 5 mg/dose every 6 hours.

Onset will occur in 15 minutes; however, maximum effects may not be seen for several hours.

Enalaprilat may be useful in the hypertensive patient at risk for cerebral hypoperfusion since the drug does not impair cerebral blood flow.

Avoid use in patients with bilateral renal artery stenosis. Adjust dose in patients with renal insufficiency.

Monitor
Blood pressure (hypotension), angioedema involving face, lips and tongue, larynx (typically within 1 to 7 days of initiation), serum creatinine (adjust dose; renal dysfunction may occur), and serum potassium (hyperkalemia).

Protect from light: no

Special considerations: none

pH: 6.5 to 7.5

Stability: clear, colorless solution; stable for 24 hours in compatible diluent

Solution compatibility: D_5W, NS, D_5LR, and D_5NS

Compatible drugs

Amikacin sulfate
Aminophylline
Ampicillin sodium
Ampicillin sodium-
    sulbactam sodium
Aztreonam
Butorphanol tartrate
Calcium gluconate
Cefazolin sodium
Cefoperazone sodium
Ceftizoxime sodium
Cetazidime
Chloramphenicol sodium
    succinate
Cimetidine HCl
Clindamycin phosphate
Dobutamine HCl
Dopamine HCl
Erythromycin lactobionate
Esmolol HCl
Famotidine
Fentanyl citrate
Filgrastim
Ganciclovir sodium
Gentamicin sulfate
Heparin sodium
Hetastarch

Hydrocortisone sodium
    succinate
Labetalol HCl
Lidocaine HCl
Magnesium sulfate
Melphalan HCl
Methylprednisolone sodium
    succinate
Metronidazole
Morphine sulfate
Nafcillin sodium
Nicardipine HCl
Nitroprusside sodium
Penicillin G potassium
Phenobarbital sodium
Piperacillin sodium
Piperacillin sodium-tazobac-
    tam sodium
Potassium chloride
Potassium phosphate
Ranitidine HCl
Teniposide
Tobramycin sulfate
Trimethoprim-sulfamethox-
    azole
Vancomycin HCl
Vinorelbine tartrate

Incompatible drugs

Amphotericin B
Cefepime HCl

Phenytoin sodium

EPINEPHRINE HYDROCHLORIDE
Adrenalin®, Parke-Davis, and other manufacturers

Methods of administration
Continuous intravenous infusion, direct intravenous injection, subcutaneous injection, and intracardiac and endotracheal injection. Intracardiac and endotracheal methods of administration are only rarely used in cardiac arrest if no other access is available.

Dosing and administration
Standard: 2 mg epinephrine/250 mL of D_5W or NS (concentrated solution: 4 mg/250 mL)

Bronchospasm, anaphylactic shock
Administer as either a direct intravenous injection or subcutaneously as 0.3 to 0.5 mg (0.3 to 0.5 mL of a 1:1000 solution) every 10 to 15 minutes. As an alternative, patients with a compromised airway or low blood pressure may receive the drug sublingually (0.5 mL of 1:1000), in a femoral or internal jugular vein (3 to 5 mL of 1:10,000), or through an endotracheal tube (3 to 5 mL of 1:10,000) if feasible. For severe reactions, an epinephrine continuous infusion has also been used in a dose of 1 to 2 mg/250 mL D_5W at a rate of 0.01 to 0.5 µg/kg/minute, titrating to blood pressure.

Refractory hypotension
Administer 1 mg in 250 mL D_5W as a continuous intravenous infusion at a rate of 0.1 to 1 µg/kg/minute.

Asystole
Administer 1 mg (10 mL of 1:10,000) intravenously over 5 to 15 seconds every 3 to 5 minutes. May increase to 2 to 5 mg every 3 to 5 minutes as necessary. The use of high-dose epinephrine (0.2 mg/kg or 7 mg) has been used, but is neither recommended nor discouraged by the American Heart Association Advanced Cardiac Life Support guidelines. If the intravenous route is not an option, other routes need to be con-

sidered. The intramuscular and subcutaneous routes are not optimal because of a poor perfusion. The drug can be given through the endotracheal route by diluting 2 to 2.5 times the intravenous dose in 10 mL of NS or distilled water.

Septic or cardiogenic shock
Initiate a continuous intravenous infusion at a rate of 1 µg/minute and titrate to 2 to 10 µg/minute according to hemodynamic response.

Endotracheal administration is 2 to 2.5 times the peripheral intravenous dose diluted in 10 mL of normal saline or sterile water for injection.

Rapid administration may cause a rapid rise in blood pressure, resulting in cerebral hemorrhage.

Monitor
Desired response (eg, resolution of heart contractions), pulmonary function, blood pressure (hypertension), heart rate (increased), chest pain, ECG (arrhythmia), urine output (decreased due to vasoconstriction), and extravasation (may result in necrosis).

Protect from light: yes (undiluted)

Special considerations:
Rate control device recommended for continuous infusions; infuse continuous infusion through central line.

pH: 2.5 to 5.0

Stability
Discard if discolored (typically pink or brown); incompatible with alkaline solutions; unstable in pH higher than 5.5; a pH of 3 to 4 is considered optimal.

Solution compatibility: D_5W, NS, and LR

Compatible drugs

Amrinone lactate
Atracurium besylate
Calcium chloride
Calcium gluconate
Diltiazem HCl
Famotidine
Heparin sodium
Hydrocortisone sodium
   succinate
Pancuronium bromide
Phytonadione
Potassium chloride
Vecuronium bromide

Incompatible drugs

Aminophylline
Amphotericin B
Ampicillin sodium
Azathioprine sodium
Ganciclovir sodium
Lidocaine HCl
Pentobarbital sodium
Phenobarbital sodium
Propofol
Sodium bicarbonate
Warfarin sodium

ERYTHROMYCIN LACTOBIONATE
various manufacturers

Methods of administration
Intermittent intravenous infusion (over 30 to 60 minutes), *not* direct intravenous injection (local irritation), and *not* intramuscular (painful on injection)

Dosing and administration
Standard: 500 mg/250 mL and 1 g/250 mL of NS

Erythromycin is a macrolide antibiotic that is active against gram-positive cocci (staphylococci and streptococci) as well as gram-positive bacilli including *Bacillus anthracis, Corynebacterium* sp, *Clostridium* sp, and *Listeria monocytogenes.* Erythromycin is also active against some gram-negative cocci *(Neisseria* sp*)* and some gram-negative bacilli, including some strains of *Haemophilus influenzae* and *Legionella pneumophila.* Some strains of *Chlamydia* sp, *Actinomyces* sp, and *Mycoplasma pneumoniae* are inhibited by erythromycin.

Treatment of skin and soft-tissue infections and infections of the respiratory tract
Administer 500 mg by intermittent intravenous infusion every 6 hours.

Treatment of Legionnaires' disease
Administer 1 g every 6 hours, then reduce to 500 mg every 6 hours after clinical response has occurred. May also be combined with rifampin for synergy. Doxycycline and ciprofloxacin are alternatives.

General
Penicillin is the treatment of choice for *Streptococcus pneumonia*e. Erythromycin is an acceptable alternative. Penicillin-resistant pneumococci may also be resistant to erythromycin.

Erythromycin is contraindicated in patients with a severe, documented allergy to it.

No dosage reduction necessary for patients with renal

insufficiency. Negligible removal of erythromycin lactobion-ate by hemodialysis. Limited data in patients with liver dys-function; dosage adjustment is generally recommended.

Monitor
Signs of infection (temperature, white blood cell count with differential), culture and susceptibility, gastrointestinal effects, ototoxicity (especially in patients with liver or renal dysfunc-tion), liver function tests (hepatic dysfunction and cholestatic jaundice have occurred), and thrombophlebitis.

Concomitant administration of erythromycin may increase plasma concentrations of theophylline, carbamazepine, cyclosporine, digoxin, and warfarin.

Concomitant administration with astemizole, terfenadine, and cisapride may result in life-threatening arrhythmia. Concomitant administration with lovastatin may result in rhabdomyolysis.

The estolate salt of erythromycin has been observed to induce hepatotoxicity in pregnant patients. In one analysis, approximately 10% of 161 patients treated with erythromycin estolate in the second trimester had elevated levels of serum glutamic-oxaloacetic transaminase. Levels returned to normal upon discontinuation of drug.

Protect from light: no

Special considerations: none

pH: 6.5 to 7.5 (with sterile water for injection)

Stability
Optimal pH is 6 to 8; solutions with a pH less than 5.5 are unstable and rapidly lose their potency; should be reconstitut-ed with sterile water for injection without preservatives to avoid gel formation. Constituted solutions are stable for 14 days in refrigeration, or for 24 hours at room temperature (sev-eral manufacturers recommend that only stable for 8 hours).

Solution compatibility: NS, D_5NS, and D_5W; (see stabili-ty section) if D_5W is used, sodium bicarbonate is added at 0.5 mL 8.4% sodium bicarbonate per 100 mL of D_5W.

Compatible drugs

Acyclovir sodium
Amiodarone HCl
Cyclophosphamide
Diltiazem HCl
Magnesium sulfate
Enalaprilat
Esmolol HCl
Famotidine
Foscarnet sodium

Heparin sodium
Hydromorphone
Labetalol HCl
Meperidine HCl
Morphine sulfate
Multivitamins
Perphenazine
Tacrolimus
Zidovudine

Incompatible drugs

Amphotericin B
Ampicillin sodium
Ascorbic acid injection
Aztreonam
Cefamandole nafate
Cefazolin sodium
Cefmetazole sodium
Cefonicid sodium
Cefotetan disodium
Cefoxitin sodium
Ceftizoxime sodium
Chloramphenicol sodium
   succinate
Dexamethasone sodium
   phosphate
Doxycycline hyclate
Fluconazole
Furosemide

Ganciclovir sodium
Ketorolac tromethamine
Metaraminol bitartrate
Metoclopramide HCl
Metoprolol tartrate
Mezlocillin sodium
Minocycline HCl
Moxalactam disodium
Nitroprusside sodium
Penicillin G potassium
Penicillin G sodium
Pentobarbital sodium
Phenobarbital sodium
Potassium chloride
Ticarcillin disodium
Ticarcillin disodium-
   clavulanate potassium

ESMOLOL HYDROCHLORIDE
Brevibloc®, Ohmeda

Methods of administration
Direct intravenous injection and continuous intravenous infusion

Dosing and administration
Standard: 2.5 g/250 mL of D_5W or NS

Supraventricular tachycardia (SVT) and hypertension
Administer 250 to 500 µg/kg direct intravenous injection over 1 minute, then administer a continuous infusion at 25 to 50 µg/kg/minute. Increase the maintenance dose by 25 µg/kg/minute every 10 to 20 minutes until desired response to a maximum of 300 µg/kg/minute. Typically, patients will respond at 50 to 200 µg/kg/minute. As the desired response is reached, the maintenance dose increment can be reduced. After discontinuation of infusion, recovery from β-blockade is observed within 10 to 20 minutes.

Dose is not altered by renal or hepatic disease.

Only the 10 mg/mL concentration in 10-mL vials is acceptable for direct intravenous injection. Other concentrations need to be diluted prior to use.

Pharmacologic effects are additive with digoxin and calcium channel blockers.

Monitor
ECG, blood pressure (hypotension), cardiac (signs and symptoms of heart failure), heart rate (bradycardia), and respiratory status (bronchospasm, wheezing, or dyspnea).

Protect from light: no

Special considerations:
Rate control device recommended for continuous infusion.

pH: 3.5 to 5.5 (concentrate); 4.5 to 5.5 (ready to use)

Stability

Relatively stable at neutral pH, with optimal stability at 3.5 to 5.5; degradation may occur with alkaline or acidic solutions; stable at room temperature for 24 hours.

Solution compatibility: D_5W, NS, and LR

Compatible drugs

Amikacin sulfate
Aminophylline
Ampicillin sodium
Atracurium besylate
Butorphanol tartrate
Calcium chloride
Cefazolin sodium
Cefoperazone sodium
Ceftazidime
Ceftizoxime sodium
Cimetidine HCl
Clindamycin phosphate
Diltiazem HCl
Dopamine HCl
Enalaprilat
Erythromycin lactobionate
Famotidine
Fentanyl citrate
Gentamicin sulfate
Heparin sodium
Hydrocortisone sodium
    succinate
Insulin, regular

Labetalol
Magnesium sulfate
Metronidazole
Midazolam
Morphine sulfate
Nafcillin sodium
Nitroglycerin
Nitroprusside sodium
Norepinephrine bitartrate
Pancuronium bromide
Penicillin G potassium
Phenytoin sodium
Piperacillin sodium
Potassium chloride
Potassium phosphate
Ranitidine HCl
Sodium acetate
Tacrolimus
Tobramycin sulfate
Trimethoprim-sulfamethox-
    azole
Vancomycin HCl
Vecuronium bromide

Incompatible drugs

Amrinone lactate
Amphotericin B
Azathioprine sodium
Cefamandole nafate
Cefotetan disodium
Chloramphenicol sodium
  succinate
Dexamethasone sodium
  phosphate
Diazepam
Furosemide
Ganciclovir sodium
Ketorolac tromethamine
Methylprednisolone sodium
  succinate
Mezlocillin
Minocycline HCl
Pentobarbital sodium
Phenobarbital sodium
Propofol

FAMOTIDINE
Pepcid®, Merck & Co., Inc.

Methods of administration
Direct intravenous injection (undiluted), intermittent intravenous infusion (over 15 to 30 minutes), and continuous intravenous infusion

Dosing and administration
Standard: 20 mg/100 mL of D_5W or NS or 40 mg/100 mL of D_5W or NS

Gastrointestinal disorders
Administer 20 mg famotidine by direct intravenous injection (may be pushed over 2 minutes) or intermittent intravenous infusion every 12 hours. For a continuous intravenous infusion, 40 mg of the drug can be diluted in 100 mL of D_5W or NS and initiated at a rate of 1.6 mg/hour. The infusion rate should be titrated to a gastric pH >4 for prophylaxis or >7 for treatment.

Famotidine has been used for prevention of stress ulceration, treatment of gastric or duodenal ulcers, and control of gastric pH in critically ill patients.

Dose or interval adjustment may be necessary in patients with renal insufficiency (creatinine clearance <50 mL/minute). Administer 50% of the dose or administer 20 mg every 24 hours. No dosage adjustment is generally required in patients with hepatic impairment.

Monitor
Symptomatic response to therapy, gastric pH, signs of bleeding (eg, occult blood), central nervous system effects (eg, headache, dizziness, confusion; mental status changes occur most frequently in elderly patients, or in patients with hepatic or renal dysfunction; probably less frequently than with cimetidine), hematologic effects (neutropenia, thrombocytopenia), and serum creatinine (monitor renal status to correct dose).

Protect from light: no

Special considerations: none

pH: 5 to 5.6 (injection); 5.7 to 6.4 (premixed)

Stability
Store in refrigerator; stable at room temperature for 48 hours in common diluents.

Solution compatibility: D_5W, NS, $D_{10}W$, and LR

Compatible drugs

Aminophylline	Epinephrine HCl
Ampicillin sodium-sulbactam sodium	Erythromycin lactobionate
	Esmolol
Ampicillin sodium	Filgrastim
Amrinone lactate	Fluconazole
Amsacrine	Fludarabine phosphate
Atropine sulfate	Folic acid
Aztreonam	Furosemide
Bretylium tosylate	Gentamicin sulfate
Calcium gluconate	Haloperidol lactate
Cefazolin sodium	Heparin sodium
Cefoperazone sodium	Hydrocortisone sodium succinate
Cefotaxime sodium	
Cefotetan disodium	Imipenem-cilastatin sodium
Cefoxitin sodium	Insulin, regular
Ceftazidime	Isoproterenol HCl
Ceftizoxime sodium	Labetolol HCl
Cefuroxime sodium	Lidocaine HCl
Cisplatin	Magnesium sulfate
Cyclophosphamide	Meperidine HCl
Dexamethasone disodium phosphate	Methotrexate sodium
	Methylprednisolone sodium succinate
Digoxin	
Dobutamine HCl	Metoclopramide HCl
Dopamine HCl	Midazolam
Enalaprilat	Morphine sulfate

Nafcillin sodium
Nitroprusside sodium
Norepinephrine bitartrate
Phenylephrine HCl
Phenytoin sodium
Phytonadione
Piperacillin sodium
Potassium chloride
Potassium phosphate

Procainamide HCl
Sargramostim
Sodium bicarbonate
Thiamine HCl
Ticarcillin disodium
Ticarcillin disodium-
    clavulanate potassium
Verapamil HCl
Vinorelbine

Incompatible drugs

Amphotericin B
Aziothioprine sodium
Cefepime HCl
Cefmetazole
Ceftriaxone sodium
Chloramphenicol sodium
    succinate

Ganciclovir sodium
Minocycline HCl
Piperacillin sodium-
    tazobactam sodium
Propofol

FENTANYL CITRATE
Sublimaze®, Akorn, Inc., and other manufacturers

Methods of administration
Intramuscular (rarely used in the intensive care setting), direct intravenous injection, continuous intravenous infusion, and epidural

Dosing and administration
Standard: 1000 μg/100 mL of D_5W or NS (concentrated solution: 50 μg/mL)

Pain control
Fentanyl can be given in a dose of 0.5 μg/kg intravenously every 1 to 2 hours. In the intensive care setting, the drug is usually given by continuous intravenous infusion at a dose of 1 to 2 μg/kg/hour after a loading dose of 1 to 2 μg/kg. Fentanyl has been administered by patient-controlled analgesia in a concentration of 10 μg/mL (basal: 0-0.14 μg/kg/hour; bolus: 0.14 μg/kg) with an 8-minute lockout period. Due to patient variability in response, titration of fentanyl to effect pain management will be required.

Morphine sulfate is the preferred analgesic for critically ill patients. Hydromorphone may be used as an alternative. Fentanyl is the preferred agent in patients with hemodynamic instability, in patients experiencing histamine release with morphine, and in patients with morphine allergy. Meperidine is generally not recommended for use because the active metabolite normeperidine may accumulate and produce central nervous system stimulation. (See practice parameters for analgesia and sedation in suggested readings.)

Dosage equivalents
fentanyl 0.1 mg = hydromorphone 1.5 mg =
  meperidine 100 mg = morphine 10 mg

If patients switch to a different analgesic or route, it is recommended that two thirds of the equianalgesic dose be given.

Fentanyl has a shorter duration of pain relief than morphine at 1 to 2 hours for a single parenteral dose. Therefore, fentanyl is usually given by continuous infusion for pain control in the intensive care setting. Because of differences in lipophillicity, an accurate conversion between fentanyl and morphine is difficult.

Transdermal fentanyl patches can be used for chronic pain (not acute pain). Maximal effects will not be seen for 24 hours after application of patch. Absorption increases with increased body temperature (eg, fever). The patch should not be altered (cut), since controlled delivery is then affected.

Fentanyl dosage should be decreased in patients with renal dysfunction. With a creatinine clearance of 10 to 50 mL/minute, give 75% of dose, and in patients with <10 mL/minute give 50% of dose.

Monitor

Pain relief, respiratory effects (use with caution in patients who are compromised, or on concomitant respiratory depressants; naloxone can be used to reverse effects), skeletal and thoracic muscle rigidity occurs more frequently following rapid intravenous administration, central nervous system effects (sedation, euphoria, pupillary constriction), physical and psychological dependence, constipation (provide stool softeners as needed), urinary retention, blood pressure (hypotension, especially with rapid infusion), and heart rate (can cause bradycardia). Use with caution in patients with existing bradycardia. Reverse with atropine.

Tolerance develops with chronic use and coincides with the development of physical dependence. Physical dependence can occur after only 2 weeks of therapy. Need to slowly taper dose over several days to minimize the effects. Signs of fentanyl withdrawal include anxiety, tachycardia, and gastrointestinal distress.

In some patients (head trauma), the pattern and degree of pain are important diagnostic indicators. Examine all appropriate alternatives.

Protect from light: yes (intact vials); not necessary after dilution for infusion

Special considerations
Use only preservative-free fentanyl when preparing epidural infusion.

pH: 4 to 7.5

Stability
Stable at room temperature after dilution for at least 48 hours; drug is hydrolyzed in acidic solutions (pH <4).

Solution compatibility: D_5W and NS

Compatible drugs

Atracurium besylate	Midazolam HCl
Enalaprilat	Nafcillin sodium
Esmolol HCl	Pancuronium bromide
Heparin sodium	Potassium chloride
Hydrocortisone sodium succinate	Sargramostim
	Vecuronium bromide
Labetolol HCl	

Incompatible drugs

Pentobarbital sodium

FLUCONAZOLE
Diflucan®, Pfizer Inc

Method of administration
Intermittent intravenous infusion (do not exceed a rate of 200 mg/hour)

Dosing and administration
Standard: 200 mg/100 mL or 400 mg/200 mL of NS or D_5W

Fluconazole is a triazole-derivative antifungal agent that is active against many fungi, including yeast and dermatophytes.

Treatment of oropharyngeal or esophageal candidiasis
Administer 200 mg intravenously on the first day, followed by 100 mg once daily.

Treatment of systemic candidiasis
Administer 400 mg intravenously the first day, followed by 200 mg to 400 mg every 24 hours.

Treatment of cryptococcal meningitis
Administer 400 mg intravenously on the first day, followed by 200 to 400 mg once daily for 10 to 12 weeks after cerebrospinal fluid culture becomes negative.

General
Same dose required for intravenous and oral administration.
Patients with a creatinine clearance of 10 to 30 mL/minute can receive 100% of the dose every 24 hours. When the creatinine clearance is less than 10 mL/minute, administer 100% of the dose every 48 hours. No dosage adjustment recommended in patients with hepatic failure. Fifty percent of fluconazole is removed by hemodialysis. Administer the usual recommended dose after each hemodialysis.

Monitor
Signs of infection (temperature, white blood cell count with differential), culture and susceptibility, liver function tests

(increase in serum transaminase levels, and hepatic necrosis), gastrointestinal effects (nausea, anorexia, and weight loss), hypersensitivity, central nervous system effects (drowsiness, headache, and insomnia), and signs of central nervous system toxicity (neuromuscular hyperirritability and convulsions).

Increases in serum drug levels of phenytoin and cyclosporine have occurred with concomitant administration of fluconazole; fluconazole may inhibit warfarin metabolism, resulting in an increase in prothrombin time response. Co-administration with terfenadine and astemizole increases risk of cardiovascular toxicity. Rifampin increases fluconazole metabolism (a higher dose of fluconazole may be needed).

Protect from light: no

Special considerations: none

pH: 4 to 8 (in sodium chloride diluent); 3.5 to 6.5 (in dextrose diluent)

Stability
Do not use if cloudy or if there is precipitate; reconstituted solutions stable at room temperature; do not refrigerate.

Solution compatibility: D_5W and NS

Compatible drugs

Acyclovir sodium	Chlorpromazine HCl
Allopurinol sodium	Cimetidine HCl
Amikacin sulfate	Dexamethasone sodium
Aminophylline	phosphate
Ampicillin sodium- sulbactam sodium	Diltiazem HCl
	Diphenhydramine HCl
Aztreonam	Dobutamine HCl
Benztropine mesylate	Dopamine HCl
Cefazolin sodium	Droperidol
Cefepime HCl	Famotidine
Cefotetan disodium	Filgrastim
Cefoxitin sodium	Fludarabine phosphate

Foscarnet sodium
Ganciclovir sodium
Gentamicin sulfate
Heparin sodium
Hydrocortisone sodium
    phosphate
Immune globulin
    intravenous
Leucovorin calcium
Melphalan HCl
Meperidine HCl
Meropenem
Metoclopramide HCl
Metronidazole
Midazolam HCl
Morphine sulfate
Nafcillin sodium
Nitroglycerin
Ondansetron HCl
Oxacillin sodium

Paclitaxel
Pancuronium bromide
Penicillin G potassium
Phenytoin sodium
Piperacillin sodium-tazobac-
    tam sodium
Prochlorperazine edisylate
Promethazine HCl
Ranitidine HCl
Sargramostim
Tacrolimus
Teniposide
Ticarcillin disodium-
    clavulanate potassium
Tobramycin sulfate
Vancomycin HCl
Vecuronium bromide
Vinorelbine tartrate
Zidovudine

Incompatible drugs

Amphotericin B
Ampicillin sodium
Calcium gluconate
Cefotaxime sodium
Ceftazidime
Ceftriaxone sodium
Cefuroxime sodium
Chloramphenicol sodium
    succinate
Clindamycin phosphate
Dantrolene sodium
Diazepam
Diazoxide

Digoxin
Erythromycin lactobionate
Furosemide
Haloperidol lactate
Hydroxyzine HCl
Imipenem-cilastatin sodium
Pentamidine isethionate
Piperacillin sodium
Propofol
Ticarcillin disodium
Trimethoprim-sulfamethox-
    azole

FLUMAZENIL
Romazicon®, Roche Pharmaceuticals

Methods of administration

Direct intravenous injection (over 30 seconds; administer through a freely flowing intravenous line in a large vein to minimize pain on injection), and intermittent intravenous infusion

Dosing and administration

Standard: 1 mg/10 mL (undiluted for direct IV injection)

Benzodiazepine-induced sedation
Administer 0.2 mg by direct intravenous injection over 15 seconds. Repeat the dose after 1 minute if desired effects are not achieved. Maximum recommended dose is 1 mg over 5 to 10 minutes.

Acute benzodiazepine overdose
Administer 0.2 mg by direct intravenous injection over 30 seconds. Administer an additional 0.3 mg dose over 30 seconds if the desired effects have not been achieved. Maximum recommended dose is 5 mg; reevaluate diagnosis of benzodiazepine overdose if no response. May need to readminister medication in 20-minute intervals. Generally not recommended for use with mixed overdoses (ie, patients using several medications) because of increased risk of seizures (especially in patients with a history of seizures or in patients using tricyclic antidepressants) and arrhythmias (bradycardia, asystole, and tachycardia).

Eighty percent of patients will respond within 5 minutes. If patients have received high doses or use benzodiazepines with long half-lives (such as diazepam), the effects of overdose may be prolonged. The effects of flumazenil may last only 1 hour; therefore, the patient must be reevaluated for the need for repeated doses of flumazenil.

Will reverse sedative, anxiolytic, anticonvulsant, anesthetic, muscle relaxant, and hypnotic effects. Flumazenil will not consistently reverse amnesia, respiratory depression, hypoventilation (need to establish airway and assist ventilation), or cardiac depression.

Monitor
Desired effects (eg, reversal of sedation), benzodiazepine withdrawal syndrome including agitation and tremors (risk in patients who have taken benzodiazepines long enough to develop a tolerance), respiratory depression/hypoventilation, cardiac depression (drug does not reverse), and seizure activity.

Several factors increase risk of seizures with the administration of this drug, including treatment of patients with long-term benzodiazepine use (increased risk of withdrawal), tricyclic antidepressant overdose, and those with a history of seizure activity or myoclonic jerking prior to administration of flumazenil.

Use with caution for patients in the intensive care unit because of unrecognized benzodiazepine dependence. Signs of withdrawal include agitation, tremors, and sensory distortion. Should not be used to reverse long-term sedation with benzodiazepine in the intensive care unit. May produce withdrawal seizures. Much better to wean the benzodiazepines gradually and allow a natural "wake up" period in the patient.

Patient should be monitored at least 3 hours after initial flumazenil administration.

Protect from light: no

Special considerations: none

pH: 4

Stability
Not generally combined with diluent; once transferred into syringe, use within 24 hours.

Solution compatibility: D_5W, NS, and LR

Drug compatibility: limited data available

FOSPHENYTOIN SODIUM
Cerebyx®, Parke-Davis

Methods of administration
Intramuscular and intermittent intravenous infusion (rate not exceeding 150 mg of phenytoin equivalent units per minute).

Dosing and administration
Standard: 1 g PE/100 mL of D_5W or NS

(Doses of 15 to 20 mg/kg for status epilepticus and 10 to 20 mg/kg in nonemergent situations are the doses in the package insert. However, most epileptologists use the higher doses because there is a greater risk to the patient if the seizures persist as compared to the risks with the elevated serum concentrations. Ample literature supports this dosing.)

Fosphenytoin is a prodrug of phenytoin with 1.5 mg of fosphenytoin administered equal to 1 mg of phenytoin produced. Fosphenytoin should be prescribed, dispensed, and administered as phenytoin equivalent units (PE). One mg PE of fosphenytoin is the equivalent of 1 mg of IV phenytoin. Fosphenytoin is packaged as 50 mg PE/mL (eg, 100 mg phenytoin = 100 mg PE fosphenytoin). Continuous EKG, blood pressure, and respiratory status monitoring are required for IV loading dose administration .

Status epilepticus and prevention and treatment of seizures during neurosurgery
Fosphenytoin should be used only for short-term parenteral administration. The loading dose is 18 to 20 mg PE/kg given intravenously at a rate of 100 to 150 mg PE/minute (over 5 to 7 minutes), or intramuscularly. Determine the patient's actual body weight in kilograms. For status epilepticus loading dose: 18 to 20 mg/kg at a rate not to exceed 150 mg PE/minute. If seizures continue, after the loading dose is completed, an additional dose of 5 mg PE/kg $\times$ 2 may be given. The nonemergent loading dose of fosphenytoin is 15 to 20 mg PE/kg given IV or IM. The initial maintenance dose is 4 to 6 mg PE/kg/day. It can also be substituted short-term for oral phenytoin dosed the

same way as the oral dose and may be given IM once daily.

For indications other than status epilepticus, fosphenytoin may be given at 50 mg to 100 mg PE/minute IV to decrease adverse reactions such as paresthesias and hypotension. IM fosphenytoin doses may be given in 1 or 2 sites regardless of dose without patient discomfort or increased risk of tissue damage.

Do not use in patients with sinus bradycardia, sino-atrial block, second- or third-degree AV block, and Adams-Stokes syndrome.

Because the effects of phenytoin as well as fosphenytoin are not immediate, concomitant administration of a benzodiazepine such as lorazepam will be necessary to control status epilepticus.

In patients with renal or hepatic insufficiency, there will be an increased fraction of unbound phenytoin. Fosphenytoin metabolic conversion to phenytoin may be increased in these patients without a similar increase in phenytoin clearance. Obtaining unbound phenytoin levels may be more helpful than measuring total phenytoin. Age, gender, and race have negligible effects on fosphenytoin pharmacokinetics.

Monitor

Seizure occurrence (primarily resolution of seizures*; both convulsive and electrographic), serum phenytoin concentration, hypotension (especially at high doses and high rates of infusion), cardiovascular effects (increased risk with hemodynamic instability, elderly, compromised pulmonary function, and co-existing cardiac arrhythmias), pruritus, respiratory function, nausea, vomiting, albumin, renal and hepatic disease (clearance to phenytoin may be increased), central nervous system effects (usually drug-concentration related and includes tremor confusion), heart rate (bradycardia, which may be dose related, and drug concentration-related effects such as nystagmus, blurred vision, drowsiness, and hyperglycemia. (See drug interactions statement in phenytoin section.)

*Continued seizures are rare

Lacks cardiovascular adverse effects associated with the propylene glycol diluent of phenytoin. Local irritation at injection site is less frequent and less severe than that seen with phenytoin preparations.

Fosphenytoin will provide 0.0037 mmol phosphate per mg of PE, which should be considered in patients with phosphate restrictions such as those with severe renal insufficiency.

Therapeutic drug monitoring considerations
(It is important to assess whether the patient is at steady state when interpreting levels.)

    Sample collection:
        Trough within 1 hour prior to dose
        Peak 3 to 4 hours after dose or loading infusion
    Therapeutic range:
        Total: 10 to 20 µg/mL
        Unbound: 1 to 2 µg/mL

Note: Do not obtain phenytoin concentrations until conversion to phenytoin is complete (2 hours after fosphenytoin infusion and 4 hours after intramuscular administration). Prior to the conversion, typical assay measurements may overestimate plasma phenytoin concentrations because of cross-reactivity with fosphenytoin.

Protect from light: no

Special considerations: none

pH: 8.6 to 9.0 undiluted

Stability
Stable in D_5W and NS for at least 30 days at room temperature.

Solution compatibility: D_5W, NS, and D_5NS

Drug compatibility
Limited data available

FUROSEMIDE
Lasix®, Hoechst Marion Roussel, and other manufacturers

Methods of administration
Intramuscular, direct intravenous injection, intermittent intravenous infusion, and continuous intravenous infusion

Dosing and administration
Standard: 40 mg/4 mL (undiluted)

Edema with left ventricular dysfunction, cirrhosis, hypercalcemia, acute pulmonary edema, oliguria, cerebral edema, and hypertension

The usual initial dose of furosemide depends on the reason for treatment and on patient response. Typically, furosemide is initiated as 20 to 40 mg by direct intravenous injection over 1 to 2 minutes. Dose can be doubled in 1 to 2 hours if no response is seen. Doses in excess of 500 mg are not likely to be effective. The effective dose is repeated twice to four times daily. Repeat as needed.

A continuous intravenous infusion of 0.25 to 0.75 mg/kg/hour may be used for patients who do not respond to a direct intravenous injection. Doses that are 200 mg or less may be given over 10 minutes. Doses that are more than 200 mg should be placed in 50 mL of D_5W or NS and administered at a rate no faster than 4 to 10 mg/minute to minimize the risk of ototoxicity.

The combination of metolazone with furosemide may result in a larger than expected increase in diuresis, as well as electrolyte loss.

Higher doses (more than 100 mg) may be necessary to initiate a response in patients with renal dysfunction. Patients using the drug for oliguria may require doses exceeding 500 mg to reach an adequate response.

Monitor
Changes in urine output, patient weight, serum electrolytes (sodium [hyponatremia], potassium [hypokalemia], chloride

[hypochloremic alkalosis], magnesium [hypomagnesemia], glucose [hyperglycemia], calcium [hypocalcemia], bicarbonate, blood urea nitrogen, and serum creatinine), intravascular volume (depletion), respiratory status, cardiovascular hemodynamics, blood pressure (hypotension), and ototoxicity (tinnitus or hearing loss).

Protect from light: yes (not required after dilution)

Special considerations: none

pH: 8 to 9.3

Stability
Do not use solutions that have a yellow color. Refrigeration may result in precipitate; however, resolubilization upon warming should not affect stability. Generally unstable in acidic media but stable in basic media.

Solution compatibility: D_5NS, $D_{10}W$, LR, and NS

Compatible drugs

Amikacin sulfate	Leucovorin calcium
Aztreonam	Melphalan HCl
Cefepime HCl	Meropenem
Cisplatin	Methotrexate sodium
Cyclophosphamide	Milrinone lactate
Cytarabine	Paclitaxel
Famotidine	Piperacillin sodium-tazobactam sodium
Fludarabine phosphate	
Fluorouracil	Tacrolimus
Foscarnet sodium	Tobramycin sulfate
Gentamicin sulfate	Vinblastine sulfate
Granisetron HCl	Vincristine sulfate
Heparin sodium	Vinorelbine tartrate
Hydrocortisone sodium succinate	

Incompatible drugs

Amrinone lactate
Amsacrine
Ascorbic acid
Atracurium besylate
Benztropine mesylate
Buprenorphine HCl
Butorphanol tartrate
Chlorpromazine HCl
Cimetidine HCl
Ciprofloxacin
Diazepam
Diltiazem HCl
Diphenhydramine HCl
Dobutamine HCl
Doxorubicin HCl
Doxycycline hyclate
Droperidol
Erythromycin lactobionate
Esmolol HCl
Fluconazole
Haloperidol lactate
Hydralazine HCl
Hydroxyzine HCl
Idarubicin HCl
Isoproterenol HCl
Labetalol HCl
Meperidine HCl
Methyldopa HCl
Metoclopramide HCl
Midazolam HCl
Minocycline HCl
Morphine sulfate
Nalbuphine HCl
Norepinephrine
Ondansetron HCl
Papaverine HCl
Pentamidine isethionate
Pentazocine lactate
Phentolamine mesylate
Prochlorperazine edisylate
Promethazine HCl
Protamine sulfate
Pyridoxine HCl
Quinidine gluconate
Thiamine HCl
Vancomycin HCl
Verapamil HCl

GENTAMICIN SULFATE
Garamycin®, Schering Corporation, and other manufacturers

Methods of administration
Intramuscular, intermittent intravenous infusion (over 30 minutes), intrathecal, and intraventricular

Dosing and administration
Standard: Dose/50 to 100 mL of NS or D_5W; larger (eg 500 mg) doses are diluted in 100 mL

Gentamicin is an aminoglycoside that is active against many aerobic gram-negative bacteria, including *Escherichia coli, Haemophilus influenzae, Moraxella lacunata, Neisseria* sp, *Proteus* sp, *Serratia* sp, and *Pseudomonas* sp (including most strains of *Pseudomonas aeruginosa*). Gentamicin is usually less active than tobramycin against *P aeruginosa*. However, gentamicin is slightly more active against *Serratia* sp and *E coli* than tobramycin. Gentamicin is active against some aerobic gram-positive bacteria, including *Staphylococcus aureus* and *Staphylococcus epidermidis*. Gentamicin is minimally active against streptococci.

Treatment of suspected or documented gram-negative infections
Administer a loading dose of 2 mg/kg total body weight (TBW) followed by a maintenance dose of 3 to 5 mg/kg in two or three divided doses (typical dose for an individual with adequate renal function [creatinine clearance greater than 70 mL/minute] is 80 mg every 8 hours). Dosage should be based on TBW and not ideal body weight (IBW). If patient is morbidly obese, then weight should be determined by using the formula IBW + 0.4 (TBW − IBW). Round to the nearest 10 mg. Pharmacokinetic monitoring is required to determine appropriate dose.
    Once-a-day aminoglycoside regimens have also been used. A dose of 4 to 6 mg/kg is administered to patients who have an estimated creatinine clearance of at least 60 mL/minute.

Subsequent doses are the same as the first. However, the interval is adjusted according to pharmacokinetic parameters to achieve a trough of less than 2 µg/mL.

Intrathecal and intraventricular administration: Administer 4 to 10 mg for the treatment of gram-negative bacillary meningitis. Typically given concurrently with systemic therapy.

Used in combination with ampicillin (or vancomycin) for treatment of infections caused by *Enterococcus faecalis.* Monotherapy generally inhibits, but does not kill, the enterococcus. Combination therapy is bactericidal.

Maintenance doses must be reduced in patients with renal insufficiency (95% of drug excreted unchanged by the kidneys). For patients with a creatinine clearance of 50 to 70 mL/minute, administer gentamicin every 12 hours. For a creatinine clearance of 30 to 50 mL/minute, administer every 18 hours. For a creatinine clearance of 15 to 30 mL/minute, give gentamicin every 24 hours. For a creatinine clearance less than 15 mL/minute, give initial dose × 1 and then dose when random level <2 µg/mL. For patients receiving hemodialysis, dose after dialysis. Obtain serum drug levels as appropriate (50% to 100% dialyzable). No dosage changes recommended in patients with hepatic failure.

Monitor

Signs of infection (temperature, white blood cell count with differential), culture and susceptibility, serum creatinine, blood urea nitrogen, fluid status (input and output), signs of ototoxicity (auditory and vestibular [tinnitus, vertigo]), and serum drug concentrations.

The risk of nephrotoxicity is dependent on several factors and includes concomitant nephrotoxic drugs, age, prolonged elevated trough concentration, hydration status, dose, and duration of treatment. Generally reversible upon drug discontinuation.

Therapeutic drug monitoring considerations

Sample collection: when patient at steady state (from 3rd to 5th dose)

Peak: 30 minutes after end of 30-minute infusion
60 minutes after intramuscular injection

Trough: within 30 minutes prior to dose

Therapeutic range:

Peak: 5 to 10 μg/mL

Trough: 0.5 to 2 μg/mL

Protect from light: no

Special considerations

If concomitant penicillin or cephalosporin use is needed, administer at least 1 hour from the gentamicin and flush tubing prior to administration. Use preservative-free preparations for intrathecal and intraventricular administration.

pH: 3 to 5.5 (intramuscular or intravenous); 3.5 to 5.5 (intrathecal or when diluted with NS)

Stability

Intrathecal injection contains no preservatives and should be used immediately; reconstituted solution stable at room temperature for 24 hours.

Solution compatibility: NS, D_5W, $D_{10}W$, and LR

Compatible drugs

Acyclovir sodium
Amiodarone HCl
Amsacrine
Atracurium besylate
Aztreonam
Ciprofloxacin
Cyclophosphamide
Diltiazem HCl
Meropenem
Enalaprilat
Esmolol HCl
Famotidine
Filgrastim
Fluconazole
Fludarabine phosphate
Hydromorphone
Insulin, regular
Labetalol HCl

Magnesium sulfate
Melphalan HCl
Meperidine HCl
Morphine sulfate
Ondansetron HCl
Paclitaxel
Pancuronium bromide

Perphenazine
Sargramostim
Tacrolimus
Teniposide
Vecuronium bromide
Vinorelbine tartrate
Zidovudine

Incompatible drugs

Allopurinol sodium
Amphotericin B
Ampicillin sodium
Azathioprine sodium
Cefoperazone sodium
Cefotetan disodium
Chloramphenicol sodium
    succinate
Dexamethasone sodium
    succinate
Dopamine HCl
Folic acid (sodium salt)

Ganciclovir sodium
Heparin sodium
Hetastarch
Idarubicin HCl
Mezlocillin sodium
Oxacillin sodium
Pentamidine isethionate
Pentobarbital sodium
Phenytoin sodium
Propofol
Ticarcillin disodium

HALOPERIDOL
Haldol®, McNeil Pharmaceutical, and other manufacturers

Methods of administration

Intramuscular, direct intravenous injection, intermittent intravenous infusion, and continuous intravenous infusion

Dosing and administration

Standard: 50 to 100 mg/50 mL of D_5W

Acute agitation and delirium

Initiate at dose of 0.5 to 2 mg (mild agitation), 5 mg (moderate agitation), or 10 mg (severe agitation) as direct intravenous injection. Repeat dose every 30 minutes (maximum of 40 mg per single dose) until adequate sedation is accomplished. The regimen can be determined by summation of the total dose required to load the patient, followed by division of this total dose into scheduled (every 6 hours) doses. Reduce dose by 25% per day every 24 to 48 hours after the initial agitation event. If inadequate response, consider the addition of concurrent benzodiazepine and/or narcotic therapy.

In cases where the drug has been used long term (more than 5 days), taper over 72 hours. For longer duration of treatment, a continuous infusion of 1 to 40 mg/hour has been used.

Note: Haloperidol is the preferred agent for the treatment of delirium in the critically ill adult. (See practice parameters for intravenous analgesia in the suggested readings.) It may also offer an advantage in patients with closed head injury because of its ability to decrease intracranial pressure. However, use caution, because continuous use for more than 72 hours may retard brain injury recovery in this population.

No dosage or interval adjustment necessary in patients with renal insufficiency.

Note: Haloperidol decanoate is a depot injection and should be given through the intramuscular, not the intravenous route.

Monitor

Sedation (usually slower than benzodiazepines), resolution of agitation and delirium, extrapyramidal symptoms, acute dystonic reactions (eg, torticollis, typically responds quickly to diphenhydramine 50 mg IV, or benztropine 2 mg IV), neuroleptic malignant syndrome (dantrolene and bromocriptine used for treatment), seizures (low compared with other neuroleptics), ECG (may cause QT prolongation and should be used with caution when given concomitantly with other agents that cause prolongation of QT interval), and blood pressure (eg, hypertension, and hypotension with intramuscular or intravenous dosing).

Protect from light: yes (undiluted)

Special considerations
Use dextrose 5% to flush line before and after administration of haloperidol.

pH: 3.0 to 3.8

Stability
Exposure to light may cause grayish-red precipitate. *Not* stable in NS; stable for at least 24 hours at room temperature.

Solution compatibility: D_5W and *not* NS

Compatible drugs

Amsacrine	Melphalan HCl
Aztreonam	Nitroglycerin
Cimetidine HCl	Norepinephrine bitartrate
Dobutamine HCl	Ondansetron HCl
Dopamine HCl	Paclitaxel
Famotidine	Phenylephrine HCl
Filgrastim	Tacrolimus
Fludarabine phosphate	Vinorelbine tartrate
Lidocaine HCl	
Lorazepam	

Incompatible drugs

Allopurinol sodium
Aminophylline
Amphotericin B
Azathioprine sodium
Bretylium tosylate
Bumetanide
Calcium chloride
Cefamandole nafate
Cefazolin sodium
Cefepime HCl
Cefmetazole sodium
Cefonicid sodium
Cefoperazone sodium
Cefotaxime sodium
Cefotetan disodium
Cefoxitin sodium
Ceftazidime
Ceftizoxime
Ceftriaxone sodium
Cefuroxime
Chloramphenicol sodium
  succinate
Clindamycin phosphate
Dexamethasone sodium
  phosphate
Diphenhydramine HCl
Epoetin alpha
Fluconazole
Folic acid
Foscarnet sodium
Furosemide
Ganciclovir sodium
Heparin sodium
Hydrocortisone sodium
  succinate
Hydroxyzine HCl
Imipenem/cilastatin sodium
Ketorolac tromethamine
Magnesium sulfate
Methicillin sodium
Methylprednisolone sodium
  succinate
Metronidazole HCl
Mezlocillin sodium
Moxalactam disodium
Nafcillin sodium
Nitroprusside sodium
Oxacillin sodium
Penicillin G potassium
Penicillin G sodium
Pentobarbital sodium
Phenobarbital sodium
Piperacillin sodium
Piperacillin sodium-
  tazobactam sodium
Potassium chloride
Sargramostim
Sodium bicarbonate
Ticarcillin disodium
Ticarcillin disodium-
  clavulanate potassium

HEPARIN SODIUM
unfractionated (various manufacturers)

Methods of administration
Subcutaneous, intermittent intravenous infusion, continuous intravenous infusion (preferred over intermittent infusion in most cases), and *not* intramuscular

Dosing and administration
Standard: 25,000 units/500 mL of D_5W or NS (minimum volume 250 mL)

For treatment of venous thromboembolic disorders (see American College of Chest Physicians [ACCP] guidelines in suggested readings)
Use a continuous intravenous infusion initiated at 80 units/kg (5000 to 10,000 units), then 18 units per kg/hour. Heparin should be continued for 5 to 10 days, and oral anticoagulation therapy should be overlapped with heparin therapy for 4 to 5 days. Measure activated partial thromboplastin time (aPTT) prior to heparin therapy, 6 to 8 hours after infusion, and 6 to 8 hours after changes in infusion rate. Adjust dose as necessary to maintain an aPTT of 1.5 to 2.5 times control (heparin level of 0.2 to 0.4 units/mL).

aPPT too low: The ACCP guidelines describe a weight-based nomogram for adjusting dosage according to the aPTT value. If aPTT is <1.2 times the control, then administer an 80 unit/kg bolus and increase infusion rate by 4 units/kg/hour. If aPTT is 1.2 to 1.5 times control, then give a 40 unit/kg/hour bolus and increase infusion rate by 2 units/kg/hour. A measurement of aPTT should be obtained in 6 hours.

aPPT too high: The ACCP guidelines describe a weight-based nomogram in which the rate is decreased 2 units/kg/hour in patients with an aPPT of 2.3 to 3 times the control. In patients with an aPPT of more than 3 times the control, the infusion should be stopped for 1 hour and the rate decreased by 3 units/kg/hour. A measurement of aPPT should be obtained in 6 hours.

For prevention of venous thromboembolism
Administer heparin 5000 units subcutaneously every 8 to 12 hours in a setting of venous stasis or following surgical procedures. It is not necessary to monitor aPTT and risk of bleeding complications is minimal.

Monitor
aPTT (at baseline, and routinely to guide subsequent dosing regimens), signs of thrombus extension and pulmonary embolism, platelet count (3 to 7 days after initiation), hemoglobin, hematocrit, and signs of bleeding (common sites for bleeding include the soft tissues, urinary tract, nose, and oropharynx).

Bovine-derived heparin is more likely to produce thrombocytopenia, and when the platelet count is less than $100,000/\mu L$, some of the ACCP guidelines recommend discontinuation of therapy.

In cases of heparin overdose, therapy depends on condition of patient. In cases of extended aPTT, heparin should be discontinued, permitting the effects to clear within a few hours. In more severe cases, treatment should include maintenance of fluid volume and replacement of clotting factors. Protamine may be necessary to neutralize heparin (see page 268).

Protect from light: no

Special considerations
Rate control device recommended for continuous infusion.

pH: 5 to 8 (premixed)

Stability
No loss of potency in 24 hours over a pH range of 3.8 to 7.6; stable at room temperature for 24 hours.

Solution compatibility: D_5W, D_5NS, D_5LR, NS, and LR

Compatible drugs

Acyclovir sodium
Allopurinol sodium
Ampicillin sodium
Ampicillin sodium-
    sulbactam sodium
Atropine sulfate
Aztreonam
Calcium gluconate
Cefazolin sodium
Cefotetan disodium
Ceftazidime
Ceftriaxone sodium
Cefuroxime
Cimetidine HCl
Cisplatin
Clindamycin phosphate
Cyanocobalamin
Cyclophosphamide
Dexamethasone sodium
    phosphate
Digoxin
Diphenhydramine
Dopamine HCl
Enalaprilat
Epinephrine HCl
Erythromycin lactobionate
Esmolol HCl
Estrogens, conjugated
Famotidine
Fentanyl citrate
Fluconazole
Fludarabine phosphate
Fluorouracil
Foscarnet sodium
Furosemide

Hydralazine HCl
Hydrocortisone sodium
    succinate
Insulin, regular
Isoproterenol
Labetalol HCl
Leucovorin calcium
Lidocaine HCl
Magnesium sulfate
Melphalan HCl
Meropenem
Methicillin sodium
Methotrexate sodium
Methylprednisolone
    sodium succinate
Metoclopramide HCl
Metronidazole
Minocycline HCl
Mitomycin
Morphine sulfate
Nafcillin sodium
Nitroglycerin
Nitroprusside sodium
Norepinephrine bitartrate
Ondansetron HCl
Oxacillin sodium
Oxytocin
Paclitaxel
Pancuronium bromide
Penicillin G potassium
Pentazocine lactate
Phytonadione
Piperacillin sodium
Piperacillin sodium-
    tazobactam sodium

Potassium chloride
Prednisolone sodium
   phosphate
Procainamide HCl
Prochlorperazine edisylate
Propranolol HCl
Ranitidine HCl
Sargramostim
Sodium bicarbonate
Streptokinase
Succinylcholine chloride

Tacrolimus
Teniposide
Ticarcillin disodium
Ticarcillin disodium-
   clavulanate potassium
Vecuronium bromide
Vinblastine sulfate
Vincristine sulfate
Vinorelbine tartrate
Zidovudine

Incompatible drugs

Alteplase
Amikacin sulfate
Amiodarone HCl
Amrinone lactate
Amsacrine
Atracurium besylate
Chlorpromazine HCl
Ciprofloxacin
Codeine phosphate
Daunorubicin HCl
Diazepam
Diltiazem HCl
Dobutamine HCl
Doxorubicin HCl
Doxycycline hyclate
Droperidol

Filgrastim
Gentamicin sulfate
Haloperidol lactate
Hyaluronidase HCl
Hydroxyzine HCl
Idarubicin HCl
Meperidine HCl
Methadone HCl
Phenytoin sodium
Promethazine HCl
Propofol
Protamine sulfate
Quinidine gluconate
Tobramycin sulfate
Vancomycin HCl

HYDROCHLORIC ACID

Method of administration
Continuous intravenous infusion

Dosing and administration
Standard: 0.1 to 0.2 N HCl solution; prepare by adding 150 mL of a 1.0 N HCl solution to 1 L of D_5W or NS (130 mEq H^+/liter); for 0.1 N HCl add 8.22 mL of 36% HCl to 1 L sterile water

Metabolic alkalemia
Initiate therapy with 0.1 to 0.2 N HCl solution as a continuous intravenous infusion at a rate of 50 and 100 mL/hour, respectively. Titrate based on arterial blood gas values (at least every 4 hours), serum electrolytes, and fluid status. Increase rate of 0.2 N HCl by increments of 10 mL/hour at 2- to 4-hour intervals to a maximum infusion rate of 10 mL/kg/hour. The amount of acid needed to correct alkalosis can be determined by the following formula:

Dose of HCl (mEq) =
$0.2 \times$ body weight (kg) $\times$ (103 − observed Cl)

Most patients with severe metabolic alkalosis appear to be safely corrected over 6 to 24 hours of infusion.

Treat underlying cause of metabolic alkalosis, including correction of fluid status and electrolyte imbalance (hypokalemia, hypochloremia, and hyponatremia); treat cause of metabolic alkalosis.

Use when rapid correction of metabolic alkalosis is necessary (acetazolamide may take several hours to achieve desired effects).

Monitor
Acid/base status (goal of decreasing arterial pH by 0.02 to 0.03 pH units every 4 hours), arterial blood gas (every 4 hours),

fluid status (input and output), electrolytes (eg, potassium, bicarbonate, magnesium, and chloride). Treatment may result in transient severe respiratory acidemia.

Protect from light: no

Special considerations
Administer in glass container; tubing should be changed every 12 hours (potential for degradation of plastic); must be administered through a central venous catheter (to reduce risk of extravasation and tissue damage).

pH: 1.10 (0.1 N HCl)

Stability: do not mix with alkaline medications

Solution compatibility: NS and D_5W

Drug compatiblity: limited data available

HYDROMORPHONE HYDROCHLORIDE
Dilaudid-HP®, Knoll Laboratories, and other manufacturers

Methods of administration
Intramuscular, subcutaneous, direct intravenous injection (dilute with 4 to 5 mL of NS and give over 2 to 5 minutes), continuous intravenous infusion, and epidural (4 mg preservative-free hydromorphone in 198 mL NS for a concentration of 0.02 mg/mL)

Dosing and administration
Standard: 20 mg/100 mL of D_5W or NS

For management of moderate to severe pain
Administer 0.5 mg subcutaneously or intravenously every 10 minutes (maximum 0.02 mg/kg), then 1 to 2 mg every 1 to 6 hours as necessary for pain control. The dose should be adjusted according to the severity of pain, underlying disease, age, and size, with doses up to 14 mg being administered. As an alternative, administer a continuous infusion (20 mg in 100 mL of D_5W or NS) at a rate of 5 µg/kg/hour to a maximum of 20 µg/kg/hour.

Epidural administration of the 0.02 to 0.05 mg/mL concentration can be given at 0.15 to 0.3 mg/hour.

Morphine sulfate is the preferred analgesic for critically ill patients. Hydromorphone may be used as an alternative. Fentanyl is the preferred agent in patients with hemodynamic instability in patients experiencing histamine release with morphine, and in patients with morphine allergy. Meperidine is generally not recommended for use because the active metabolite normeperidine may accumulate and produce central nervous system stimulation. (See practice parameters for analgesia and sedation in suggested readings.)

Dosage equivalents
fentanyl 0.1 mg = hydromorphone 1.5 mg = meperidine 100 mg = morphine 10 mg

If patients switch to a different analgesic or route, it is recommended that two thirds of the equianalgesic dose be given. Hydromorphone has a shorter duration of pain relief than morphine and will require more frequent dosing. Due to differences in lipophillicity, an accurate conversion between fentanyl and hydromorphone is difficult. Dosage adjustment required for patients with hepatic impairment.

Monitor

Pain relief, respiratory effects (use with caution in patients who are compromised, or on concomitant respiratory depressants), central nervous system effects (sedation, euphoria, pupillary constriction), physical and psychological dependence, constipation (provide stool softeners as needed), urinary retention, and blood pressure (hypotension, especially with rapid infusion).

Tolerance develops with chronic use and coincides with the development of physical dependence. Physical dependence can occur after only 2 weeks of therapy. Need to slowly taper dose over several days to minimize the effects. Signs of withdrawal include anxiety, tachycardia, and gastrointestinal distress.

In some patients (head trauma), the pattern and degree of pain are important diagnostic indicators. Examine all appropriate alternatives.

Protect from light: no

Special considerations

Use only preservative-free hydromorphone when preparing epidural infusion.

pH: 4 to 5.5

Stability

A slightly yellowish color has not been associated with loss of potency. Refrigeration results in crystallization (resolubilization occurs upon warming); stable at room temperature for at least 24 hours.

Solution compatibility: D_5W, NS, D_5 $1/2$NS, D_5NS, and $1/2$NS

Compatible drugs

Acyclovir sodium
Amikacin sulfate
Ampicillin sodium
Aztreonam
Cefazolin sodium
Cefepime HCl
Cefoperazone sodium
Cefotaxime sodium
Cefotetan disodium
Cefoxitin sodium
Ceftazidime
Ceftizoxime sodium
Cefuroxime sodium
Cisplatin
Clindamycin phosphate
Cyclophosphamide
Doxycycline hyclate
Erythromycin lactobionate

Filgrastim
Gentamicin sulfate
Magnesium sulfate
Metronidazole
Mezlocillin sodium
Nafcillin sodium
Ondansetron HCl
Penicillin G potassium
Pentobarbital
Piperacillin sodium
Piperacillin sodium-
    tazobactam sodium
Ticarcillin disodium
Tobramycin sulfate
Trimethoprim-sulfamethox-
    azole
Vancomycin HCl
Vinorelbine

Incompatible drugs

Dexamethasone sodium
    phosphate
Diazepam
Minocycline HCl
Pentobarbital

Phenobarbital sodium
Phenytoin sodium
Sargramostim
Sodium bicarbonate

IMIPENEM-CILASTATIN SODIUM
Primaxin®, Merck & Co., Inc.

Methods of administration
Intramuscular (separate preparation for intramuscular use) and intermittent intravenous infusion (over 30 to 60 minutes)

Dosing and administration
Standard: 500 mg/100 mL of NS

Imipenem-cilastatin is a broad-spectrum carbapenem antibiotic. It is generally active against the following gram-positive cocci: penicillinase- and nonpenicillinase-producing strains of *Staphylococcus aureus*, *Staphylococcus epidermidis*, *Streptococcus pneumoniae*, *Streptococcus pyogenes*, *Streptococcus agalactiae*, and viridans streptococci. The drug is only bacteriostatic against enterococci.

Imipenem-cilastatin is also active against many aerobic gram-negative bacteria, such as the Enterobacteriaceae, including *Citrobacter diversus, Citrobacter freundii, Enterobacter cloacae, Enterobacter aerogenes, Escherichia coli, Hafnia alvei, Klebsiella oxytoca, Klebsiella pneumoniae, Morganella morganii, Proteus mirabilis, Proteus vulgaris, Serratia marcescens, Salmonella* sp, and *Shigella* sp.

Imipenem-cilastatin is active against many strains of *Pseudomonas aeruginosa,* including some strains resistant to third-generation cephalosporins, aminoglycosides, and extended- spectrum penicillins. It is also active against *Acinetobacter* sp and *Branhamella catarrhalis,* Imipenem-cilastatin is active against most gram-positive anaerobic bacteria including *Actinomyces* sp, *Clostridium* sp, *Peptostreptococcus* sp, and *Propionibacterium* sp. It is also active against gram-negative anaerobic bacteria, including most strains of *Bacteroides* sp, *Fusobacterium* sp, and *Veillonella* sp.

Indicated for serious infections caused by susceptible organisms including bone and joint, bacterial septicemia, intra-abdominal, lower respiratory tract, gynecologic, and skin and skin structure infections
Administer imipenem 500 mg to 1 g every 6 to 8 hours depending on the severity of the infection.

Dose or interval adjustment required for renal insufficiency (creatinine clearance less than 30 mL/minute). For patients with a creatinine clearance of 10 to 30 mL/minute, increase the dosing interval to every 8 to 12 hours. For a creatinine clearance less than 10 mL/minute, administer 500 mg every 12 to 24 hours. Administer dose after hemodialysis (20% to 50% removed). No dosage adjustment is generally recommended for patients with hepatic failure.

Monitor

Signs of infection (temperature, white blood count with differential), culture and susceptibility, hypersensitivity, hypotension and nausea (have been associated with rapid infusion), eosinophilia, gastrointestinal effects (nausea, diarrhea, vomiting), central nervous system effects (drowsiness, headache, and insomnia) and signs of toxicity (neuromuscular hyperirritability and convulsions).

Imipenem is contraindicated for use in patients with a severe, documented allergy to carbapenem antibiotics. Imipenem should be used cautiously in patients with allergies to penicillins or cephalosporins, as cross reactivity may exist.

Protect from light: no

Special considerations

If concomitant aminoglycoside use is needed, administer at least 1 hour from the imipenem-cilastatin and flush tubing prior to administration.

pH: 6.5 to 7.5

Stability

Constituted solutions are colorless to yellow. Solutions should be discarded if they darken to brown. Deterioration is concentration dependent. Stability in NS is maintained for 10 hours at room temperature, or for 48 hours under refrigeration.

Solution compatibility

D_5W (4 hours at room temperature); $D_{10}W$ (4 hours at room temperature), and NS (10 hours at room temperature)

Compatible drugs

Acyclovir sodium
Aztreonam
Cefepime HCl
Diltiazem HCl
Famotidine
Filgrastim
Fludarabine phosphate
Foscarnet sodium
Idarubicin HCl

Insulin, regular
Melphalan HCl
Methotrexate sodium
Ondansetron HCl
Procainamide
Tacrolimus
Teniposide
Vinorelbine tartrate

Incompatible drugs

Allopurinol sodium
Aminophylline
Amrinone lactate
Azathioprine sodium
Calcium chloride
Calcium gluconate
Ceftriaxone sodium
Chlorpromazine HCl
Dobutamine HCl
Fluconazole
Ganciclovir sodium
Haloperidol lactate
Mannitol
Metaraminol bitartrate

Methoxamine HCl
Midazolam HCl
Minocycline HCl
Nalbuphine HCl
Nitroprusside sodium
Pentamidine isethionate
Pentazocine lactate
Phenobarbital sodium
Prochlorperazine edisylate
Promethazine HCl
Pyridoxine HCl
Sargramostim
Sodium bicarbonate
Thiamine HCl

IMMUNE GLOBULIN, INTRAVENOUS (HUMAN) 5%
Gamimune N®, Bayer Corporation, various manufacturers

Methods of administration
Intermittent intravenous infusion and intramuscular

Dosing and administration
Depends on manufacturer

	Maximum concentration (%)	Initial infusion rate	Maximum infusion rate
Gamimune N®	10	0.01-0.02 mL/kg/min	0.08 mL/kg/min
Gammagard®	10	0.5 mL/kg/h	4 mL/kg/h
Gammar®	5	0.01-0.02 mL/kg/min	0.06 mL/kg/min
Polygam®	10	0.5 mL/kg/h	4 mL/kg/h
Sandoglobulin®	12	0.01-0.03 mL/kg/min	2.5 mL/min

Acquired immunodeficiency syndrome
Administer either 200 to 250 mg/kg every 2 weeks or 400 to 500 mg/kg every month.

Adjuvant to severe cytomegalovirus infections
Administer 500 mg/kg every other day for seven doses.

Autoimmune hemolytic anemia
Administer 500 mg/kg for 5 days. Administer booster doses as needed.

Chronic idiopathic thrombocytopenic purpura
Administer either 400 mg/kg/day for 5 days or 1 g/kg/day for

2 days; continue therapy every 3 to 6 weeks depending on clinical response. (Syndrome typically defined as a platelet count less than 100,000 in the absence of cause such as disease or toxic exposure.)

Chronic inflammatory demyelinating polyneuropathy
Administer doses of 400 mg/kg/day once each month.

Chronic lymphocytic leukemia
Administer 400 mg/kg/dose every 3 weeks.

Guillain-Barré syndrome
Administer either 400 mg/kg/day for 4 to 5 days, or 1000 mg/kg/day for 2 days, or 2000 mg/kg for 1 day.

Idiopathic thrombocytopenic purpura
Administer either 400 mg/kg/day for 5 consecutive days or 800 mg/kg/day for 2 consecutive days.

Immune mediated neutropenic disorders
Administer 400 mg/kg/dose daily for 5 days. Maintenance doses are administered as necessary.

Kawasaki disease
Administer either 400 mg/kg/day for 4 days within 10 days of onset of fever, or 800 mg/kg/day for 1 to 2 days within 10 days of onset of fever, or 2 g/kg for one dose.

Postallogeneic bone marrow transplant
Administer 500 mg/kg for 2 to 7 days before transplantation, then 500 mg/kg/week for 3 to 4 months posttransplantation.

Posttransfusion purpura
Administer 400 mg/kg/dose daily for 2 to 6 days.

Primary immunodeficiency disorders
Administer 200 to 400 mg/kg as a loading dose, then 100 to 200 mg/kg every 4 weeks. May be increased to 800 mg/kg every week if required.

Prophylaxis of infection in solid-organ transplant patients
Administer 500 mg/kg within 48 hours of organ transplanta-

tion, then 250 mg/kg weekly for 5 to 10 weeks after transplantation. (Use in CMV-seronegative recipients of CMV-seropositive organs.)

Refractory dermatomyositis
Administer 2 g/kg/dose every month for three to four doses.

Refractory polymyositis
Administer 1 g/kg/day for 2 days every month for four doses.

Monitor
Desired response (eg, increased platelets, prevention or duration of infection), mild hip, chest or back pain, hypotension, chills, fever, headache, malaise, myalgia, and dyspnea. Most adverse effects are associated with rapid infusion and typically resolve with temporary discontinuation or by decreasing the rate of infusion. Similarly, pretreatment with antihistamines (diphenhydramine 50 mg intravenously or orally), acetaminophen (650 mg orally), or dexamethasone may be helpful, but is not necessary in all patients. Refer to table for recommended initial and maximum infusion rates. Aseptic meningitis with severe headaches has been reported with high-dose immunoglobulin therapy.

The risk of transmission of either HIV or hepatitis B virus is negligible. Since 1985, potential blood donors are screened and excluded from the donor pool if they carry antibodies to HIV. The Cohn-Oncley fractionation method is used in the preparation of immunoglobulin products, which removes greater than 10^{15} units/mL of HIV by partition and inactivation of the virus. Potential donors are also screened for the presence of hepatitis B surface antigen, and units that test positive for this marker are discarded. Because of contamination of immunoglobulin products with hepatitis C, in 1994 the manufacturing process was changed. The CDC claims that products manufactured through this new process should provide negligible risk for HCV transmission to recipients.

Protect from light: no

Special considerations: none

Stability

Depends on manufacturer: refrigerate Gamimune N® and Gammagard®; Gammar®, Polygam®, and Sandoglobulin® can be stored at room temperature.

Solution compatibility: D$_5$W, NS (depends on manufacturer)

	pH	Osmolality* (based on IVIG concentration)	
Gamimune- N®	4.3 to 5	5% 10%	305 274
Gammagard®	6.8	5% 10%	636 1250
Gammar-IV®	7.0	5%	330
Polygam®	6.8	5% 10%	636 1250
Sandoglobulin®	6.0	3% NS 3% SWI 6% NS 6% SWI 12% NS 12% SWI	498 192 690 384 1074 768

*Needs to be taken into account in choosing an appropriate IVIG formulation for a patient with renal dysfunction because of difficulty in handling large osmotic load.

Compatible drugs

Fluconazole
Sargramostin

Incompatible drugs

Limited data available

INSULIN HUMAN INJECTION
Humulin®, Eli Lilly and Company, and
other manufacturers

Methods of administration
Subcutaneous, intramuscular injection, direct intravenous injection (administered over 1 to 3 seconds), and continuous intravenous infusion

Dosing and administration
Standard: 100 units regular insulin/100 mL of NS

Hyperglycemia (associated with diabetic ketoacidosis)
Initiate insulin therapy with 0.1 units/kg by direct intravenous injection, followed by a continuous intravenous infusion of 0.1 unit/kg/hour. Generally desirable to decrease blood glucose at rate of 80 to 100 mg/dL/hour. Too rapid a decrease may lead to complications including cerebral edema. Increase rate of infusion by increments of 0.1 unit/kg/hour every 2 to 4 hours, regularly checking blood glucose, acetone, and ketones. In some adults, 20,000 units in 24 hours have been required.

Concurrent infusion of D_5NS should be initiated when blood glucose falls to 250 mg/dL. Administration of dextrose with NS is recommended because the fall in glucose is usually more rapid than the resolution of ketoacidosis. At this time, the insulin infusion rate should also be decreased to 1 to 3 units/hour to maintain blood glucose at 150 to 250 mg/dL. After normalization of anion gap, subcutaneous regular insulin based on a sliding scale can be administered. Discontinue the insulin infusion 1 hour after the first subcutaneous dose.

Therapy for diabetic ketoacidosis typically consists of restoration of volume (should be given within 1 hour of initiation of treatment; may require at least 5 L of fluid), electrolyte management, reversal of acidosis and ketosis, and control of blood glucose.

For hyperglycemia associated with sepsis, diabetes, or parenteral nutrition

Administer insulin intravenously or subcutaneously with dosing based on a sliding scale (every 6 hours) or as a low-dose continuous intravenous infusion with dosing based on blood glucose levels (every 3 to 6 hours).

Only regular insulin is appropriate for intravenous use.

Dosage adjustment generally required in patients with renal insufficiency (creatinine clearance <50 mL/minute). For patients with a creatinine clearance of 10 to 50 mL/minute, administer 75% of dose. For a creatinine clearance of less than 10 mL/minute, administer 50% of dose. Insulin is not eliminated by hemodialysis or peritoneal dialysis.

Monitor

Blood and urine glucose, weight, serum and urine ketones, fluid status (input and output), electrolytes (serum sodium and potassium every 2 hours, and serum magnesium, calcium, and phosphate every 4 hours), serum creatinine, blood urea nitrogen, respiration (hyperventilation secondary to respiratory acidosis), arterial blood gases, heart rate, and blood pressure.

Nonselective β-blockers (eg, propranolol) may delay recovery and mask the signs and symptoms of hypoglycemia. Medications that may increase the hypoglycemic effect of insulin include alcohol, α-adrenergic blockers, fenfluramine, and tetracyclines. Medications that decrease the hypoglycemic effects include corticosteroids, diltiazem, dobutamine, epinephrine, and thiazide diuretics.

Signs of hypoglycemia include tachycardia, anxiety, tremors, headache, and motor dysfunction (administer glucagon or glucose).

Insulin allergies are generally secondary to species composition, but patients may be allergic to protamine. Reactions range from local erythema and pruritus to anaphylactic-type reactions.

Protect from light: no (avoid direct sunlight)

Special considerations
Prime the intravenous tubing with 20 mL of insulin solution prior to initiation of treatment (insulin adheres to containers and to plastic infusion lines). Only regular insulin may be administered intravenously; requires use of infusion pump.

pH: 7 to 7.8

Stability
Discoloration, turbidity, or unusual viscosity indicates deterioration. Refrigerate; intact vials can remain at room temperature for several months.

Solution compatibility: NS and D_5NS

Compatible drugs

Amiodarone HCl
Ampicillin sodium
Ampicillin sodium-sulbactam sodium
Aztreonam
Cefazolin sodium
Cefoperazone
Cefotetan disodium
Digoxin (NS)
Dobutamine HCl
Esmolol HCl
Famotidine
Gentamicin sulfate
Heparin sodium
Imipenem-cilastatin sodium
Magnesium sulfate
Meperidine HCl
Meropenem
Methylprednisolone sodium succinate
Midazolam HCl
Morphine sulfate
Nitroglycerin
Nitroprusside sodium
Oxytocin
Pentobarbital
Potassium chloride
Ritodrine HCl
Sodium bicarbonate
Tacrolimus
Terbutaline sulfate
Ticarcillin disodium
Ticarcillin disodium-clavulanate potassium
Tobramycin sulfate
Vancomycin HCl

Incompatible drugs

Aminophylline
Amrinone lactate
Butorphanol tartrate
Cefoperazone sodium
Cefoxitin sodium
Chlorpromazine HCl
Cytarabine
Diltiazem
Diphenhydramine HCl
Dopamine HCl
Hydroxyzine HCl
Isoproterenol HCl
Labetalol HCl

Minocycline HCl
Nafcillin sodium
Norepinephrine bitartrate
Pentamidine isethionate
Phentolamine mesylate
Phenylephrine HCl
Phenytoin sodium
Prochlorperazine edisylate
Propranolol HCl
Protamine sulfate
Quinidine gluconate
Vasopressin

ISOPROTERENOL HYDROCHLORIDE

Isuprel®, Sanofi Winthrop Pharmaceuticals, and other manufacturers

Methods of administration

Direct intravenous injection (1 mL of the 1:5000 solution should be diluted to 10 mL with NS or D_5W to provide a solution containing 20 µg/mL), continuous intravenous infusion, subcutaneous, intracardiac (in emergencies)

Dosing and administration

Standard: 2 mg/500 mL of D_5W or NS (4 µg/mL) (concentrated 4 mg/250 mL of D_5W)

Heart block and atropine-refractory bradycardia: Initiate at 2 µg/minute as an initial continuous infusion and titrate by 2 to 4 µg/minute at 5-minute intervals until asymptomatic heart rate is achieved (maintain at 2 to 20 µg/minute). No more than 10 µg/minute is necessary in most cases.

Route of administration	Preparation of dilution	Initial dose	Subsequent dose
Direct IV injection	Dilute 1 mL (0.2 mg) to 10 mL with NS or D_5W	0.02 to 0.06 mg (1 to 3 mL of USP, diluted solution	0.01 to 0.2 mg (0.5 to 10 mL of diluted solution
Continuous IV infusion	Dilute 2 mg in 500 mL of D_5W USP	2 µg/min (1.25 mL of diluted solution/min	Titrate gradually to 10 to 20 µg/min, until a heart rate of 60 beats/min
Intramuscular	Use solution 1:5000 undiluted	0.2 mg (1 mL)	0.02 to 1 mg (0.1 to 5 mL)
Subcutaneous	Use solution 1:5000 undiluted	0.2 mg (1 mL)	0.15 to 0.2 mg (0.75 to 1 mL)
Intracardiac	Use solution 1:5000 undiluted	0.02 mg (0.1 mL)	

For symptomatic bradycardia, atropine, pacing, dopamine, or epinephrine should be tried first.

Monitor
Blood pressure (hypotension), heart rate (tachycardia), angina, arrhythmias (may be exacerbated in patients with hypokalemia, hyperkalemia, acidosis, or hypercapnia).

Protect from light: yes, not necessary when diluted

Special considerations
Use filter needle when withdrawing solution from ampules; infuse through central line if possible; rate control device recommended for continuous intravenous infusion

pH: 3.5 and 4.5

Stability
Brownish pink color has developed on exposure to extreme temperatures, light, or air. Do not use if color or precipitate is present. Unstable at pH > 6; stable at room temperature

Solution compatibility: D_5W, NS, LR, and $D_{10}W$

Compatible drugs

Amiodarone HCl	Hydrocortisone sodium
Amrinone lactate	succinate
Atracurium besylate	Pancuronium bromide
Bretylium tosylate	Potassium chloride
Famotidine	Tacrolimus
Heparin sodium	Vecuronium bromide

Incompatible drugs

Aminophylline	Insulin, human
Amphotericin B	Pentobarbital sodium
Azathioprine sodium	Phenobarbital sodium
Furosemide	Sodium bicarbonate
Ganciclovir sodium	

KETOROLAC TROMETHAMINE
Toradol®, Roche Laboratories Inc.

Methods of administration
Intramuscular, direct intravenous injection (over at least 15 seconds), and intermittent intravenous infusion

Dosing and administration
Typically given by intramuscular or direct intravenous injection. If given by intermittent intravenous infusion, 30 mg ketorolac/50 mL of D_5W or NS is used.

Short-term maintenance of pain
Administer 30 to 60 mg, then 15 to 30 mg every 6 hours as needed, not to exceed 120 mg in a 24-hour period. It is not recommended to be used for more than 5 days.

Not recommended to use in patients with renal insufficiency; however, if needed, dose and interval adjustment required in patients with a creatinine clearance less than 50 mL/minute.

Monitor
Pain relief, inflammation, gastrointestinal effects (peptic ulceration and bleeding), renal status (alters the autoregulation of renal blood flow; may cause renal insufficiency, acute renal failure, and interstitial nephritis; dosage adjustment is recommended), and signs of bleeding.

Co-administration with lithium will increase lithium serum levels.

Adjust dose in patients with renal insufficiency (50% of dose should be used in geriatric patients and patients with renal insufficiency). Generally not necessary to alter dose in patients with liver impairment, however, use with caution.

Protect from light: yes (injection)

Special considerations: none

pH: 6.9 to 7.9

Stability

Precipitation may occur at low pH values; admixture stable for 48 hours at room temperature.

Solution compatibility: D_5W, NS, D_5NS, and LR

Compatible drugs

Limited data available

Incompatible drugs

Amrinone lactate
Amphotericin B
Azathioprine sodium
Calcium chloride
Chlorpromazine HCl
Cisatracurium besylate
Diazepam
Diphenhydramine HCl
Dobutamine HCl
Doxycycline hyclate
Erythromycin lactobionate
Esmolol HCl
Ganciclovir sodium
Haloperidol lactate
Hydroxyzine HCl

Labetalol HCl
Metaraminol bitartrarte
Midazolam HCl
Minocycline HCl
Nalbuphine HCl
Pentamidine isethionate
Pentazocine lactate
Pentobarbital
Phentolamine mesylate
Prochlorperazine edisylate
Promethazine HCl
Protamine sulfate
Pyridoxine HCl
Quinidine gluconate
Vancomycin HCl

LABETALOL HYDROCHLORIDE
Normodyne®, Schering Corporation, and other manufacturers

Methods of administration
Direct intravenous injection, and continuous intravenous infusion

Dosing and administration
Standard: 200 mg/200 mL of D_5W or NS

Severe hypertension and hypertensive emergencies
For use as a direct intravenous injection, administer 10 to 20 mg over 2 minutes. Escalating doses of 20 to 40 mg may be administered at 10-minute intervals (up to a maximum of 300 mg) to achieve desired response.

For use as a continuous intravenous infusion, initiate at a rate of 2 mg/minute and titrate according to response. Usual effective dose is 50 to 200 mg (maximum cumulative dose recommended is 300 mg over 24 hours).

A continuous infusion is prepared by adding 2 ampules (100 mg × 2) to 160 mL of D_5W to yield a final concentration of 1 mg/mL.

Following intravenous administration, the maximal effect occurs within 5 to 10 minutes and typically persists for at least 6 hours. Elderly patients may achieve a greater reduction in blood pressure at lower doses.

Labetalol does not significantly reduce cerebral blood flow and therefore is useful in patients with cerebrovascular disease. Because of its beta-blocking properties, the drug should not be used in patients with asthma, sinus bradycardia, severe heart failure, or heart block greater than first degree, and it should be used cautiously in patients with intermittent claudication and Raynaud's phenomenon. Labetalol may mask symptoms of hypoglycemia in patients with insulin-dependent diabetes mellitus.

The presence of renal insufficiency should not necessitate dose adjustment. Labetalol is predominantly eliminated by glucuronidation in the liver with less than 5% excreted unchanged. Dosage adjustment may be necessary in hepatic impairment.

Monitor

Blood pressure (eg, hypotension), signs and symptoms of heart failure, respiratory status (eg, bronchospasm, wheezing, and dyspnea), dose-related drowsiness, paresthesias, and heart rate (bradycardia).

Labetalol should not be administered within 2 hours of a calcium channel blocker (AV conduction abnormalities and myocardial contractility depression).

Protect from light: yes (not diluted solution)

Special considerations:

Use filter needle for ampules; rate control device recommended for continuous infusion.

pH: 3.0 to 4.0

Stability

Solution is clear and colorless to slightly yellow; precipitation occurs in alkaline solutions; most stable at pH of 2 to 4.

Solution compatibility: D_5W, NS, D_5LR, D_5NS, and LR

Compatible drugs

Amikacin sulfate	Cimetidine HCl
Aminophylline	Clindamycin phosphate
Amiodarone HCl	Dobutamine HCl
Ampicillin sodium	Dopamine HCl
Butorphanol tartrate	Enalaprilat
Calcium gluconate	Erythromycin lactobionate
Cefazolin sodium	Esmolol HCl
Ceftazidime	Famotidine
Ceftizoxime sodium	Fentanyl citrate
Chloramphenicol sodium succinate	Gentamicin sulfate
	Heparin sodium

Lidocaine HCl
Magnesium sulfate
Meperidine HCl
Metronidazole
Midazolam HCl
Morphine sulfate
Nitroglycerin
Nitroprusside sodium
Norepinephrine bitartrate
Oxacillin sodium
Penicillin G potassium
Piperacillin sodium
Potassium chloride
Potassium phosphate
Ranitidine HCl
Tobramycin sulfate
Trimethoprim-sulfamethox-
    azole
Vancomycin HCl

Incompatible drugs

Amphotericin B
Azathioprine sodium
Cefmetazole sodium
Cefonicid sodium
Cefoperazone sodium
Cefotaxime sodium
Cefotetan disodium
Cefoxitin sodium
Ceftriaxone sodium
Cefuroxime sodium
Dexamethasone sodium
    phosphate
Furosemide
Hydrocortisone sodium
    succinate
Insulin, human
Ketorolac tromethamine
Methicillin sodium
Mezlocillin sodium
Moxalactam disodium
Nafcillin sodium
Penicillin G sodium
Propofol
Sodium bicarbonate

LIDOCAINE HYDROCHLORIDE
Xylocaine®, Astra USA, Inc., and other manufacturers

Methods of administration
Intramuscular, continuous intravenous infusion, and direct intravenous injection

Dosing and administration
Standard: 2 g/500 mL of D_5W or NS (4 mg/mL) (concentrated: 2 g/250 mL)

Ventricular arrhythmias including tachycardia, fibrillation, and PVCs associated with myocardial infarction or angina
Initiate with a direct intravenous injection of 1 to 1.5 mg/kg at a rate no faster than 50 mg/minute. May repeat at doses of 1 to 1.5 mg/kg in 3 to 5 minutes up to a total dose of 3 mg/kg.

A continuous intravenous infusion of 60 to 120 µg/kg/minute may be initiated over 20 minutes. Patients can be typically maintained on 15 to 30 µg/kg/minute (2 to 4 mg/minute). Slower infusion rates may be initiated for patients with congestive heart failure or liver disease, or those receiving cimetidine or β–blockers. Endotracheal dose is 2 to 2.5 times the intravenous dose. The drug should be diluted in 10 mL of either NS or distilled water.

Reduce dose 50% in patients with acute hepatitis or cirrhosis.

Monitor
ECG (arrhythmias), mental status (confusion, hallucinations, psychosis, especially with prolonged infusions), convulsions (may require diazepam for treatment), blood pressure (eg, hypotension), and thrombophlebitis (patients receiving prolonged infusions).

Therapeutic drug monitoring considerations
Sample collection:
Obtain 6 to 12 hours after initiation of therapy
Therapeutic range:
1.5 to 5.0 µg/mL

Toxicity usually causes central nervous system effects such as dizziness, drowsiness, paresthesias, convulsions, and visual disturbances. Cardiovascular toxicity typically occurs when lidocaine serum concentrations exceed 9 µg/mL. Phenobarbital and phenytoin may increase lidocaine clearance, thereby lowering lidocaine serum concentration.

Protect from light: no

Special considerations: rate control device recommended

pH: 3.5 to 6 (premixed solution) or 5 to 7 (syringes)

Stability: stable at room temperature; expiration data on premixed bag or for 30 days out of wrapper; pH for maximum stability is 3 to 6.

Solution compatibility: D_5W (preferred diluent), NS, LR, $D_5^{1/2}NS$, D_5NS

Compatible drugs

Alteplase	Haloperidol lactate
Amiodarone HCl	Heparin sodium
Amrinone lactate	Labetalol HCl
Cefazolin sodium	Meperidine HCl
Ciprofloxacin	Morphine sulfate
Diltiazem HCl	Nitroglycerin
Dobutamine HCl	Nitroprusside sodium
Dopamine HCl	Potassium chloride
Enalaprilat	Streptokinase
Famotidine	

Incompatible drugs

Amphotericin B	Norepinephrine bitartrate
Ampicillin sodium	Pentobarbital sodium
Azathioprine sodium	Phenobarbital sodium
Epinephrine HCl	Phenytoin sodium
Ganciclovir sodium	Propofol
Isoproterenol HCl	

LORAZEPAM
Ativan®, Wyeth-Ayerst Laboratories

Methods of administration
Intramuscular (administered deep into muscle mass), direct intravenous injection (dilute with equal amount of D_5W and administer over 1 minute [2 mg/minute] directly into a vein or into the tubing of a running intravenous infusion), and intermittent intravenous infusion

Dosing and administration
Standard: 20 mg/100 mL of D_5W or NS. (Concentrations up to 100 mg/100 mL have been used in volume-restricted patients or if precipitation is a problem.)

Agitation, anxiety, sedation, and amnesia
Initiate therapy at 0.5 to 1 mg for mild and 2 to 4 mg for moderate to severe agitation as a direct intravenous injection. Repeat with a dose of 1 to 2 mg if inadequate response after 10 minutes. Consider alternative or concurrent therapy if no response. Lorazepam is the preferred agent for prolonged treatment of anxiety in the critical care patient. (See practice parameters for intravenous analgesia and sedation in suggested readings.)

When given as an intravenous injection, a rate not exceeding 2 mg/mL should be used. When administering lorazepam by continuous infusion, a bolus dose should be given prior to each increase in infusion rate.

Status epilepticus
Initiate with 4 mg by direct intravenous injection. Repeat with same dose every 10 to 15 minutes as necessary, as tolerated, up to a maximum 10 mg in 1 hour. Typically, phenytoin, fosphenytoin, or phenobarbital is initiated to control seizures in the long term.

Taper the dose for patients getting prolonged therapy (eg, more than 7 days) over 72 hours to avoid withdrawal. Withdrawal effects include tremors, diaphoresis, irritability, and insomnia.

Compared with midazolam, lorazepam causes less hypotension, more rapid awakening, equal degree of anterograde amnesia, and at a lower cost. Dosage or interval adjustment not necessary in patients with renal or hepatic insufficiency.

Monitor

Seizure control, sedation, agitation, respiratory effects (especially with concomitant medications that cause respiratory depression, including narcotics), blood pressure (decrease in blood pressure with rapid administration and in patients with hypovolemia, hyperthermia, and vasoconstriction), physical dependence (potential with chronic use), tolerance (develops in response to the nonanxiolytic actions of lorazepam, not the anxiolytic effects; leads to severe withdrawal if drug is stopped abruptly), respiratory depression, paradoxical central nervous system effects including excitation, agitation, and delirium (especially in the elderly).

Protect from light: yes (undiluted)

Special considerations

Avoid intra-arterial administration of benzodiazepines because it may produce spasm, along with gangrene that may require intervention.

pH: N/A (not in aqueous base)

Stability

Do not use if discolored or contains precipitate. Refrigerate for storage, but may remain at room temperature for up to 2 weeks. Lorazepam must be diluted immediately prior to injection with an equal volume of compatible diluent. Some clinicians have commented on precipitation problems occurring more frequently with different IV pumps.

Solution compatibility: D_5W (preferred as diluent) and NS

Compatible drugs

Acyclovir sodium
Allopurinol sodium
Amsacrine
Atracurium besylate
Cefepime HCl
Cisplatin
Cyclophosphamide
Diltiazem HCl
Doxorubicin HCl
Filgrastim
Fludarabine phosphate
Haloperidol lactate
Melphalan hydrochloride
Paclitaxel
Pancuronium bromide
Piperacillin sodium-
    tazobactam sodium
Tacrolimus
Teniposide
Vecuronium bromide
Vinorelbine tartrate
Zidovudine

Incompatible drugs

Aztreonam
Buprenorphine HCl
Idarubicin HCl
Ondansetron HCl
Propofol
Sargramostim

MAGNESIUM SULFATE
various manufacturers

Methods of administration
Intramuscular, intermittent intravenous infusion, and continuous intravenous infusion

Dosing and administration
Standard: 1 to 2 g/50 mL or 3 to 4 g/100 mL of D_5W or NS; maximum intravenous concentration 200 mg/mL; intramuscular administration 500 mg/mL

Hypomagnesemia
Identify and eliminate the causes of hypomagnesemia including renal (eg, hypercalcemia, osmotic diuresis), loop diuretics, aminoglycosides, and amphotericin B, or gastrointestinal losses (eg, diarrhea, malnutrition, and nasogastric suctioning).

Administer 1 to 2 g of magnesium sulfate over 1 hour for moderate (magnesium levels of 1 to 1.7 mg/dL), and 3 to 4 g over 2 hours for severe, symptomatic hypomagnesemia (serum magnesium concentrations typically less than 1 mg/dL). For patients with mild to moderate hypomagnesemia, delivery of magnesium sulfate over longer periods of time (6 to 8 hours) may optimize magnesium retention. In moderate hypomagnesemia, the 1-g dose may be repeated every 6 to 12 hours. For severe hypomagnesemia, more sustained doses may be required. An additional 2 g should be administered every 4 hours for two doses, then 1 g every 6 hours, as needed.

Preeclampsia/seizure prophylaxis
Initiate with 4 g of magnesium sulfate over 1 hour followed by a continuous intravenous infusion of 1 g/hour (20 g magnesium sulfate in 500 mL of D_5W or NS). A maximum dose of 2.5 g/hour.

Refractory ventricular tachycardia or fibrillation
Administer 2 g by direct intravenous administration. (For refractory ventricular tachycardia infuse over 3 to 5 minutes. For ventricular fibrillation administer intravenous push.) fol-

lowed by a continuous infusion of 1 g/hour for 24 hours.

$$1 \text{ g} = 8 \text{ mEq elemental magnesium}$$
$$1 \text{ mmol/L} = 2 \text{ mEq} = 24 \text{ mg elemental magnesium}$$

Accumulation occurs in patients with renal insufficiency and end-stage renal disease. Doses may need to be more conservative (eg, 50% of dose) in this patient population.

Monitor
Signs and symptoms of hypomagnesemia: hyperexcitability, hyperactive reflexes, muscle twitching, central nervous system effects (confusion, agitation, seizures), ECG changes (flattened T waves and prolonged QT intervals), cardiovascular effects (decrease in cardiac output, supraventricular and ventricular tachycardia).

Other monitoring parameters: Magnesium serum concentrations (obtain at least 1 hour after administration of magnesium; reference range for adults of 1.5 to 2.5 mg/dL; hypoalbuminemia and hemodilution may give a low total serum magnesium concentration with active ionized concentrations being adequate), electrolytes (hypomagnesemia often causes hypokalemia and hypocalcemia), and hypotension and flushing (with too rapid an infusion).

Complications may occur secondary to hypermagnesemia. Signs and symptoms include depressed central nervous system, diarrhea, flushing, and depression of deep tendon reflexes. Hypermagnesemia can be treated with calcium gluconate.

Protect from light: no

Special considerations: none

pH: 5.5 to 7.0

Stability
Insoluble with phosphates, alkali carbonates, and bicarbonates; stable at room temperature for 60 days.

Solution compatibility: D_5W

Compatible drugs

Acyclovir sodium
Amikacin sulfate
Ampicillin sodium
Aztreonam
Cefazolin sodium
Cefoperazone sodium
Cefotaxime sodium
Cefoxitin sodium
Chloramphenicol sodium
   succinate
Dobutamine HCl
Doxycycline hyclate
Enalaprilat
Erythromycin lactobionate
Esmolol HCl
Famotidine
Gentamicin sulfate
Heparin sodium
Hydrocortisone sodium
   succinate
Hydromorphone HCl

Idarubicin HCl
Insulin, regular
Labetalol HCl
Meperidine HCl
Meropenem
Metronidazole (ready
   to use)
Minocycline HCl
Morphine sulfate
Nafcillin sodium
Ondansetron HCl
Penicillin G potassium
Piperacillin sodium
Piperacillin sodium-
   tazobactam sodium
Potassium chloride
Ticarcillin disodium
Tobramycin sulfate
Trimethoprim-
   sulfamethoxazole
Vancomycin HCl

Incompatible drugs

Aminophylline
Amphotericin B
Amrinone lactate
Azathioprine sodium
Calcium chloride
Cefepime HCl
Ceftriaxone sodium
Cefuroxime sodium
Ciprofloxacin
Clindamycin phosphate
Cyclosporine

Dexamethasone sodium
   phosphate
Dobutamine
Haloperidol lactate
Methylprednisolone sodium
   succinate
Mezlocillin sodium
Pentamidine isethionate
Phytonadione
Sodium bicarbonate
Tetracycline

MANNITOL
various manufacturer

Methods of administration
Intermittent intravenous infusion or continuous infusion

Dosing and administration
Standard: 100 g/500 mL of D_5W (20% solution)

Acute intracranial hypertension
Initiate therapy with 0.5 to 1 g/kg as a 20% to 25% solution over 30 to 60 minutes. Maintenance doses of 0.25 to 0.5 g/kg by intermittent intravenous infusion over 15 minutes every 4 to 6 hours are used. Alternatively, the drug can be administered by continuous intravenous infusion as a 20% solution at a rate of 10 to 20 mL/hour. Slowly taper over 3 to 4 days to decrease risk of rebound increases in intracranial pressure.

Diuresis
Initiate therapy at 50 to 100 g daily (12.5 to 25 g every 6 hours) as a 15% to 20% solution over at least 90 minutes by intermittent intravenous infusion.

Patients with congestive heart failure or pulmonary edema may benefit from premedication with furosemide.

Monitor
Fluid status (dehydration secondary to diuresis; fluid input and output), serum osmolality (obtain every 12 hours; goal of 310 to 320 mOsm/kg or at least 10 mOsm/L above baseline), intracranial pressure, cerebral perfusion pressure (MAP-ICP), complications of volume expansion (eg, congestive heart failure and pulmonary edema), electrolytes (potassium, sodium, and magnesium), and renal status.

Protect from light: no

Special considerations
Administer through an in-line 5 micron filter set for concentrations >20%.

pH: 4.5 to 7

Stability
Incompatible with strongly acidic and basic solutions; store at room temperature.

Solution compatibility: D_5W, NS, and D_5NS, LR

Compatible drugs

Allopurinol sodium	Ondansetron HCl
Aztreonam	Paclitaxel
Fludarabine phosphate	Piperacillin sodium-
Fluorouracil	tazobactam sodium
Gallium	Sargramostim
Idarubicin HCl	Tenoposide
Melphalan	Vinorelbine tartrate

Incompatible drugs

Amrinone lactate	Filgrastim
Cefepime HCl	Imipenem-cilastatin sodium
Cisplatin	Potassium chloride

MEPERIDINE HYDROCHLORIDE
Demerol®, Sanofi Winthrop Pharmaceuticals, and other manufacturers

Methods of administration
Intramuscular, subcutaneous, direct intravenous injection (10 mg/mL concentration given slowly), and intermittent intravenous infusion

Dosing and administration
Standard: 10 mg/mL

For moderate to severe pain
Administer 25 to 100 mg intravenously every 3 or 4 hours as necessary.

Morphine sulfate is the preferred analgesic for critically ill patients. Hydromorphone may be used as an alternative. Fentanyl is the preferred agent in patients with hemodynamic instability, in patients experiencing histamine release with morphine, and in patients with morphine allergy. Meperidine is generally not recommended for use because the active metabolite normeperidine may accumulate and produce central nervous system stimulation. (See practice parameters for analgesia and sedation in the suggested readings.)

Dosage equivalents
fentanyl 0.1 mg = hydromorphone 1.5 mg = meperidine 100 mg = morphine 10 mg

If patients switch to different analgesics or route, it is recommended that two thirds of the equianalgesic dose be given. Meperidine has a shorter duration of pain relief than morphine.

Because of the potential for seizures with the accumulation of the meperidine metabolite (normeperidine), many clinicians will not use this drug in patients with decreased renal function.

If the drug is used, dosage and interval adjustments are necessary in patients with a creatinine clearance less than 50 mL/minute secondary to accumulation of metabolite.

Administer 75% of the dose to patients with a creatinine clearance of 10 to 50 mL/minute. Contraindicated in patients with end-stage renal disease.

Monitor

Pain relief, respiratory effects (use with caution in patients who are compromised or on concomitant depressants), central nervous system effects (sedation, euphoria, pupillary constriction), allergic reactions (some products contain sulfites), physical and psychological dependence, constipation (provide stool softeners as needed), urinary retention, blood pressure (hypotension, especially with rapid infusion), and serum creatinine (normeperidine may accumulate and cause twitching, tremors, or seizures).

Tolerance develops with chronic use and coincides with the development of physical dependence. Physical dependence can occur after only 2 weeks of therapy. Need to slowly taper dose over several days to minimize the effects. Signs of withdrawal include anxiety, tachycardia, and gastrointestinal distress.

In some patients (head trauma), the pattern and degree of pain are important diagnostic indicators. Examine all appropriate alternatives.

Protect from light: yes (vials)

Special considerations: none

pH: 3.5 to 6

Stability: stable at room temperature

Solution compatibility: D_5W, NS, $D_{10}W$, R, LR, and 1/2NS

Compatible drugs

Acyclovir sodium
Amikacin sulfate
Ampicillin sodium
Ampicillin sodium-
    sulbactam sodium
Atenolol
Aztreonam
Bumetanide
Cefazolin sodium
Cefotaxime sodium
Cefotetan disodium
Cefoxitin sodium
Ceftazidime
Ceftizoxime sodium
Ceftriaxone sodium
Cefuroxime sodium
Chloramphenicol sodium
    succinate
Clindamycin phosphate
Dexamethasone sodium
    phosphate
Digoxin
Diltiazem HCl
Diphenhydramine HCl
Dobutamine HCl
Dopamine HCl
Doxycycline hyclate
Droperidol
Erythromycin lactobionate
Famotidine
Filgrastim
Fluconazole
Fludarabine phosphate
Gentamicin sulfate

Hydrocortisone sodium
    succinate
Insulin, regular
Labetalol HCl
Lidocaine HCl
Magnesium sulfate
Methylprednisolone sodium
    succinate
Metoclopramide HCl
Metoprolol tartrate
Metronidazole
Ondansetron HCl
Oxacillin sodium
Oxytocin
Paclitaxel
Penicillin G sodium
Penicillin G potassium
Piperacillin sodium
Piperacillin sodium-
    tazobactam sodium
Potassium chloride
Propranolol HCl
Ranitidine HCl
Sargramostim
Teniposide
Ticarcillin disodium
Ticarcillin disodium-
    clavulanate potassium
Tobramycin sulfate
Trimethoprim-
    sulfamethoxazole
Vancomycin HCl
Verapamil HCl
Vinorelbine

Incompatible drugs

Aminophylline
Amphotericin B
Azathioprine sodium
Cefamandole nafate
Cefepime HCl
Cefmetazole sodium
Cefonicid sodium
Cefoperazone sodium
Diazepam
Furosemide
Ganciclovir sodium
Heparin sodium
Idarubicin HCl
Imipenem-cilastatin sodium
Methicillin sodium
Mezlocillin sodium
Minocycline HCl
Morphine sulfate
Nafcillin sodium
Pentobarbital sodium
Phenobarbital sodium
Phenytoin sodium
Propofol
Sodium bicarbonate

MEROPENEM
Merrem®, Zeneca Pharmaceuticals

Methods of administration
Direct intravenous injection (administer into a vein or into the tubing of a freely flowing compatible intravenous solution over 3 minutes) and intermittent intravenous infusion (over 15 to 30 minutes)

Dosing and administration
Standard: 500 mg/50 mL and 1 g/100 mL of NS or D_5W

Meropenem is a broad-spectrum carbapenem antibiotic that is generally active against the following gram-positive aerobic cocci: penicillinase- and nonpenicillinase-producing strains of *Staphylococcus aureus, Staphylococcus epidermidis, Streptococcus pneumoniae, Streptococcus pyogenes, Streptococcus agalactiae,* and viridans streptococci. The drug is only bacteriostatic against enterococci. Meropenem is also active against many aerobic gram-negative bacteria, such as the Enterobacteriaceae, including *Citrobacter diversus, Citrobacter freundi, Enterobacter cloacae, Enterobacter aerogenes, Escherichia coli, Hafnia alvei, Klebsiella oxytoca, Klebsiella pneumoniae, Morganella morganii, Proteus mirabilis, Proteus vulgaris, Serratia marcescens, Salmonella* sp, and *Shigella* sp.

Meropenem is active against many strains of *Pseudomonas aeruginosa,* including some strains resistant to third-generation cephalosporins, aminoglycosides, and extended-spectrum penicillins. It is also active against *Acinetobacter* sp and *Branhamella catarrhalis.* Meropenem is active against most gram-positive anaerobic bacteria including *Actinomyces* sp, *Clostridium* sp, *Peptostreptococcus* sp, and *Propionibacterium* sp. It is also active against gram-negative anaerobic bacteria, including most strains of *Bacteroides* sp, *Fusobacterium* sp, and *Veillonella* sp.

Meropenem is more active in vitro than imipenem-cilastatin against Enterobacteriaceae and less active against gram-positive bacteria.

Indicated for mixed infections usually requiring antibiotic combinations (eg, intra-abdominal infections, pulmonary infections) and infections caused by multiresistant gram-negative pathogens, including Pseudomonas aeruginosa *and* Enterobacteriaceae.

Administer 1 g every 8 hours.

Dosage or interval adjustment required for patients with renal insufficiency (creatinine clearance less than 50 mL/minute). For patients with a creatinine clearance of 25 to 50 mL/minute, increase interval to every 12 hours. For a creatinine clearance of 10 to 25 mL/minute, administer 50% of the dose every 12 hours. For a creatinine clearance less than 10 mL/minute, administer 50% of the dose every 24 hours. For patients receiving hemodialysis, give the maintenance dose after dialysis. No dosage adjustment in patients with hepatic dysfunction.

Monitor

Signs of infection (temperature, white blood cell count with differential), culture and susceptibility, liver function tests, gastrointestinal effects (nausea, diarrhea, and vomiting), eosinophilia, central nervous system effects (drowsiness, headache, and insomnia), hypersensitivity, and signs of toxicity (ataxia, dyspnea, and convulsions). Meropenem does not have the epileptogenic potential that is seen with imipenem-cilastatin.

Meropenem is contraindicated for use in patients with a severe, documented allergy to carbapenem antibiotics. Meropenem should be used cautiously in patients with allergies to penicillin or cephalosporin antibiotics, as cross-reactivity may exist.

Protect from light: no

Special considerations

If concomitant aminoglycoside use is needed, administer at least 1 hour from meropenem and flush tubing prior to administration.

pH: 7.3 to 8.3 (constituted)

Stability
Constituted solution varies from colorless to yellow depending on the concentration. Stability in NS is maintained for 4 hours at room temperature, or for 24 hours under refrigeration. Stability in D_5W is maintained for 1 hour at room temperature, or for 4 hours under refrigeration.

Compatible drugs

Aminophylline	Furosemide
Atropine sulfate	Gentamicin sulfate
Atenolol	Heparin sodium
Cimetidine HCl	Insulin, regular
Dexamethasone sodium	Magnesium sulfate
phosphate	Metoclopramide HCl
Digoxin	Metronidazole
Diphenhydramine HCl	Morphine sulfate
Dobutamine HCl	Norepinephrine bitartrate
Dopamine HCl	Phenobarbital sodium
Doxycycline hyclate	Ranitidine HCl
Enalaprilat	Vancomycin HCl
Fluconazole	

Incompatible drugs

Acyclovir sodium	Doxycycline hyclate
Calcium gluconate	Ondansetron HCl
Diazepam	Zidovudine

METHYLPREDNISOLONE SODIUM SUCCINATE

Solu-Medrol®, Pharmacia & Upjohn Company, and other manufacturers

Methods of administration

Intramuscular, direct intravenous injection (doses up to 125 mg/dose over 3 to 15 minutes), intermittent intravenous infusion (over 15 to 60 minutes), and continuous intravenous infusion

Dosing and administration

Standard: Dose/50 mL of D_5W or NS; larger doses (eg 9 grams) are diluted in 500 mL; 500 mg over 2 to 5 minutes

Spinal cord injury
Administer an initial dose of 30 mg/kg in 50 mL NS by intravenous injection over 15 minutes, followed by 5.4 mg/kg/hour for 23 hours. Some data suggests that this rate be continued for 48 hours. Administer within 8 hours of acute spinal cord injury.

Status asthmaticus
Administer 2 mg/kg/day in three to four divided doses for 48 hours, then 60 to 80 mg/day until PEF reaches 70% of predicted or personal best. Typically administered for 3 to 10 days. If patients are initiated on corticosteroids, it is not necessary to taper the corticosteroid dose, unless continued for more than 7 days.

General
Guidelines from the National Heart, Lung, and Blood Institute suggest that there is no advantage in using higher doses of corticosteroids in severe asthma exacerbations, nor is there an advantage in using intravenous over oral therapy in most patients.

Dosage or interval adjustments are generally not required in patients with renal insufficiency.

Monitor

Desired effects, signs of infection (may also mask signs of infection; corticosteroids may mask fever or cause leukocytosis), fluid status, serum glucose (glucose intolerance), impaired wound healing, electrolytes (eg, potassium, sodium), acid/base status (metabolic alkalosis), and central nervous system effects (eg, psychosis, depression, euphoria).

Phenobarbital and phenytoin may reduce serum methylprednisolone concentrations and may impair the therapeutic effects.

Hypotension, cardiac arrhythmias, and sudden death have been reported with high doses (>500 mg) over < 20 minutes.

Protect from light: no

Special considerations: none

pH: 7 to 8 (reconstituted solution)

Stability

Intact vials stored at room temperature; admixtures stable at room temperature for at least 48 hours.

Solution compatibility: D_5W, NS, D_5NS, and LR

Compatible drugs

Acyclovir sodium
Amrinone lactate
Aztreonam
Cefepime HCl
Cisplatin
Cyclophosphamide
Cytarabine
Doxorubicin HCl
Enalaprilat
Famotidine
Fludarabine phosphate
Heparin sodium
Insulin, regular
Melphalan HCl
Meperidine HCl
Methotrexate sodium
Morphine sulfate
Piperacillin sodium-
    tazobactam sodium
Potassium chloride (D_5W)
Sodium bicarbonate
Tacrolimus
Teniposide

Incompatible drugs

Allopurinol
Amphotericin B
Ampicillin sodium
Ampicillin sodium-
    sulbactam sodium
Amsacrine
Azathioprine sodium
Calcium chloride
Calcium gluconate
Cefmetazole sodium
Cefotaxime sodium
Cefoxitin sodium
Ciprofloxacin
Diltiazem HCl
Diphenhydramine HCl
Doxycycline hyclate
Esmolol HCl (D_5W)
Filgrastim
Ganciclovir sodium
Haloperidol lactate
Hydralazine HCl
Magnesium sulfate
Metaraminol bitartrate
Minocycline HCl
Nafcillin sodium
Nalbuphine HCl
Ondansetron HCl
Paclitaxel
Papaverine HCl
Penicillin G sodium
Pentamidine isethionate
Pentazocine lactate
Potassium chloride
Promethazine HCl
Propofol
Protamine sulfate
Pyridoxine HCl
Quinidine gluconate
Sargramostim
Thiamine HCl
Vinorelbine tartrate

METOCLOPRAMIDE HYDROCHLORIDE
Reglan®, A. H. Robins Company, and other manufacturers

Methods of administration
Intramuscular, direct intravenous injection (undiluted over 1 to 2 minutes) and intermittent intravenous infusion

Dosing and administration
Standard: 10 mg/2 mL (undiluted if by direct IV injection)

Gastrointestinal diseases (reflux esophagitis, gastroparesis)
Administer 10 mg by slow intravenous injection up to four times daily 30 minutes prior to meals and at bedtime. Doses exceeding 10 mg need to be administered in 50 mL of D_5W or NS over 15 minutes.

For small-bowel intubation or radiological examination
Administer 10 mg/2 mL by direct intravenous injection slowly over 1 to 2 minutes.

Dose or interval adjustment necessary in patients with renal insufficiency (creatinine clearance <50 mL/minute). Administer 75% of the dose in patients with a creatinine clearance of 10 to 50 mL/minute or 50% of the dose in patients with a creatinine clearance <10 mL/miunte.

Monitor
Resolution of symptoms or other desired effects (intubation of the small intestine), sedation, extrapyramidal reactions (eg, acute dystonic reactions), gastrointestinal effects (eg, diarrhea), and serum creatinine (monitor renal status to adjust dose).

Protect from light: yes (undiluted)

Special considerations: none

pH: 3 to 6.5 (variable depending on product)

Stability
Generally stable in a pH range of 2 to 9; stable for at least 24 hours at room temperature.

Solution compatibility: D_5W, NS, $D_5^{1/2}NS$, and LR

Compatible drugs

Acyclovir sodium
Aztreonam
Ciprofloxacin
Cisplatin
Cyclophosphamide
Cytarabine
Diltiazem HCl
Doxorubicin HCl
Droperidol
Famotidine
Filgrastim
Fluconazole
Fludarabine phosphate
Foscarnet sodium
Heparin sodium
Idarubicin Hcl
Leucovorin calcium

Melphalan HCl
Meperidine HCl
Meropenem
Methotrexate sodium
Morphine sulfate
Ondansetron HCl
Paclitaxel
Piperacillin sodium-
    tazobactam sodium
Sargramostim
Tacrolimus
Teniposide
Vinblastine sulfate
Vincristine sulfate
Vinorelbine tartrate
Zidovudine

Incompatible drugs

Ampicillin sodium
Amphotericin B
Amsacrine
Amrinone lactate
Calcium gluconate
Cefepime HCl
Chloramphenicol sodium
    succinate

Erythromycin lactobionate
Fluorouracil
Furosemide
Ganciclovir sodium
Propofol
Sodium bicarbonate

METOPROLOL TARTRATE
Lopressor®, Ciba Geneva Pharmaceuticals

Methods of administration
Direct intravenous injection and intermittent intravenous infusion

Dosing and administration
Standard: 5 mg/50 mL of D_5W

Myocardial infarction
Treatment of the early phase of acute myocardial infarction should begin with the direct intravenous injection of 5 mg of metoprolol over 2 to 5 minutes for three doses (15 mg total). Oral therapy should then be initiated. However, if necessary, metoprolol can be administered by intermittent intravenous infusion as 5 mg in 50 mL over 15 to 30 minutes every 6 hours. Titrate dose based on heart rate and blood pressure.

Long-acting β-blockers and intravenous calcium channel blockers should not be administered within 2 hours of one another. Avoid abrupt withdrawal of long-term metoprolol therapy. Sudden withdrawal may precipitate or cause angina.

Monitor
ECG, heart rate, cardiac output, blood pressure, and breath sounds (bronchospasm)

Protect from light: yes (undiluted vials)

Special considerations: none

pH: approximately 7.5

Stability: stored at room temperature

Solution compatibility: D_5W and NS

Compatible drugs

Alteplase
Meperidine HCl
Morphine sulfate

Incompatible drugs

Amphotericin B
Erythromycin lactobionate

METRONIDAZOLE
Flagyl®, SCS Pharmaceuticals, and other manufacturers

Method of administration
Intermittent intravenous infusion (over 60 minutes)

Dosing and administration
Standard: 500 mg/100 mL of NS (no more than 8 mg/mL)

In general, metronidazole is active against most obligately anaerobic bacteria and many protozoa. Metronidazole is active against many anaerobic gram-negative bacilli including *Bacteroides fragilis.* The drug is also active against many aerobic gram-positive cocci such as *Clostridium* sp, including *Clostridium difficile* (oral), and *Peptostreptococcus.* It is considered the treatment of choice for infections caused by *B fragilis.* Clindamycin, cefotetan, cefmetazole, and ceftizoxime have good activity, but not to the same extent as metronidazole.

Metronidazole is active against several protozoan parasites including *Trichomonas vaginalis, Giardia lamblia,* and *Entamoeba histolytica.*

Treatment of abdominal and pelvic infections, and osteomyelitis and other infections due to susceptible anaerobic bacteria and protozoa
Administer 500 mg every 8 hours.

Dose and frequency adjustment generally not needed in patients with renal insufficiency. Parent compound and active metabolite are more than 50% removed by hemodialysis; administer dose after dialysis. Dosage adjustment probably not necessary in patients with mild hepatic failure; modify dose for severe liver failure (modify dosing interval to every 12 hours).

Monitor
Signs of infection (temperature, white blood cell count with differential), and gastrointestinal disturbances (nausea, vomiting, and metallic taste), urine color (may be slightly red

dish-brown), central nervous system effects (eg, headache, ataxis, and vertigo), and alcohol use (may cause disulfiram-type reaction; patient at risk for at least 24 hours after discontinuing medication).

Concomitant administration can cause an increase in phenytoin and lithium serum concentrations, and can cause an increase in the effects of warfarin (prolongation of PT).

Protect from light: yes

Special considerations:
None; stable for 96 hours at room light after reconstitution.

pH: 5 to 7 (ready-to-use bags, and after reconstitution)

Stability
Use reconstituted solution within 24 hours when stored at room temperature.

Solution compatibility: D_5W, NS, and LR

Compatible drugs

Acyclovir sodium	Magnesium sulfate
Allopurinol sodium	Melphalan HCl
Amiodarone HCl	Meperidine HCl
Cefepime HCl	Meropenem
Cyclophosphamide	Morphine sulfate
Diltiazem HCl	Perphenazine
Enalaprilat	Piperacillin sodium-tazobactam sodium
Esmolol HCl	
Fluconazole	Procainamide HCl
Foscarnet sodium	Sargramostim
Heparin sodium	Tacrolimus
Hydromorphone HCl	Teniposide
Labetalol HCl	Vinorelbine tartrate

Incompatible drugs

Amphotericin B
Amrinone lactate
Ascorbic acid
Aztreonam
Buprenorphine HCl
Calcium chloride
Cefamandole nafate
Cefotaxime sodium
Ceftriaxone sodium
Chlorpromazine HCl
Diphenhydramine HCl
Dobutamine HCl
Dopamine HCl
Filgrastim
Ganciclovir sodium
Haloperidol lactate
Hydroxyzine HCl
Midazolam HCl
Minocycline HCl
Ondansetron HCl
Papaverine HCl
Promethazine HCl
Quinidine gluconate
Verapamil HCl

MIDAZOLAM HYDROCHLORIDE
Versed®, Roche Pharmaceuticals

Methods of administration
Intramuscular (deep), direct intravenous injection, intermittent intravenous infusion, and continuous intravenous infusion

Dosing and administration
Standard: 100 mg/100 mL of D_5W or NS (concentrated solution: 50 mg/100 mL)

Sedation, anxiolytic, amnesia (eg, mechanically ventilated patients)
Initiate therapy at 1 to 2 mg for mild agitation (or in debilitated patients), and 2.5 to 5 mg for moderate to severe agitation as a direct intravenous injection over 1 minute. May repeat dose every 10 minutes to maximum of 20 mg. If maintenance therapy is required, midazolam may be administered as a continuous intravenous infusion at 0.5 to 10 mg/hour. Titrate at 30-minute intervals by 1.0 mg as needed for desired response (maximum: 15 mg/hour). Remember to give a partial bolus of 0.5 to 1 mg prior to increasing the infusion rate. Consider addition of narcotics or haloperidol if inadequate response.

Sedation (and to decrease anxiety and patient's memory) with procedures
Administer 1 to 2 mg as a direct intravenous injection over 2 to 3 minutes. Repeat every 5 minutes until desired effects are achieved (maximum: 5 mg cumulative dose). Debilitated patients may require lower doses (eg, 0.5 mg).

During acute agitation phase, higher doses of midazolam may be necessary to achieve desired effect, while smaller doses may maintain the desired degree of sedation once the patient has been calmed.

If patients require long-term therapy (more than 7 days), the dose should be tapered over 72 hours to minimize risk of withdrawal.

Midazolam (or propofol) is preferred for short-term treatment of anxiety in the critically ill adult. (See practice parameters for intravenous analgesia and sedation in suggested readings.) Advantage over diazepam is short half-life and brief clinical effects.

If there is a pain component to the agitation, combination therapy with a narcotic may be warranted. If narcotics or other central nervous system depressants are administered concomitantly, the midazolam may need to be reduced. Lower doses may also be necessary in the elderly.

Dose or interval adjustment needed in patients with severe renal insufficiency. When the creatinine clearance is less than 10 mL/minute, the dose should be reduced by 50%. The accumulation of metabolites may explain prolonged sedation in patients with renal failure. Because midazolam is eliminated primarily by hepatic metabolism, the dose should be reduced in patients with hepatic dysfunction.

Monitor
Sedation, respiratory effects (respiratory depression, especially when given concomitantly with other depressant drugs, including narcotics), ECG, blood pressure (hypotension may occur with aggressive loading doses or in patients who are hypovolemic, hypothermic, or have vasoconstriction), tolerance (may occur with nonanxiolytic actions with long-term therapy; does not occur with anxiolytic effects), anterograde amnesia (loss of recall of events occurring after drug; occurs more frequently than with diazepam), paradoxical central nervous system effects including delirium and agitation (especially in the elderly), and withdrawal symptoms. Has been associated with respiratory and cardiac arrest. Signs of withdrawal include tremors, diaphoresis, irritability, and insomnia.

Protect from light: yes (when diluted and stored as recommended, protection from light is not necessary)

Special considerations
Avoid intra-arterial administration of benzodiazepines because this may produce spasm, with gangrene that may require intervention.

pH: approximately 3

Stability
Colorless to light yellow solution; reportedly stable at pH of 3 to 3.6 stable for 24 hours at room temperature.

Solution compatibility: D_5W, NS, and LR (4 hours)

Compatible drugs

Amiodarone HCl
Atracurium besylate
Cisatracurium
Dopamine HCl
Esmolol HCl
Famotidine
Fentanyl citrate
Fluconazole

Insulin, regular
Labetalol HCl
Morphine sulfate
Nitroglycerin
Nitroprusside sodium
Norepinephrine bitartrate
Pancuronium bromide
Vecuronium bromide

Incompatible drugs

Aminophylline
Amphotericin B
Ampicillin sodium
Ampicillin sodium-
    sulbactam sodium
Ascorbic acid
Azathioprine
Bumetanide
Cefmetazole sodium
Cefonicid
Cefoperazone
Ceftazidime
Cefuroxime sodium
Chloramphenicol
    sodium succinate
Clindamycin phosphate
Clonidine
Dexamethasone sodium
    phosphate

Epoetin alpha
Foscarnet sodium
Furosemide
Ganciclovir sodium
Imipenem-cilastatin
    sodium
Ketorolac tromethamine
Methotrexate sodium
Metronidazole HCl
Pentobarbital sodium
Perphenazine
Phenobarbital sodium
Prochlorperazine edisylate
Propofol
Quinidine (NS)
Ranitidine HCl
Sodium bicarbonate

MORPHINE SULFATE
various manufacturers

Methods of administration
Intramuscular, subcutaneous, direct intravenous injection, intermittent intravenous infusion, continuous intravenous infusion, intrathecal, and epidural

Dosing and administration
Standard: 100 mg/100 mL or a concentrated solution of 500 mg/250 mL of D_5W or NS frequently used for continuous infusion or for patient-controlled analgesia

For moderate to severe pain, and pain of myocardial infarction
Administer 0.05 mg/kg intravenously over 10 minutes; redose every 1 to 2 hours as needed. For continuous treatment, typically more than one loading dose may be required. For maintenance, administer 2.5 to 20 mg/dose intramuscularly, subcutaneously, or intravenously every 2 to 6 hours as needed; typical dose is 10 mg/dose every 4 hours as needed.

Intramuscular is preferred over subcutaneous administration when repeat injections are necessary because of the local tissue irritation, pain, and induration associated with repeat injections using the subcutaneous route. However, the intravenous route is frequently preferred in the intensive care unit. For continuous intravenous infusion, 0.8 to 10 mg/hour is typically administered, but higher doses may be required depending on relief of pain and side effects.

Considered the drug of choice after a myocardial infarction and to treat pulmonary edema because morphine induces modest venodilation (which decreases preload), and has modest arterial vasodilating and vasotonic effects that decrease heart rate. Caution should be used in patients with inferior myocardial infarction since morphine may induce profound hypotension in these patients.

Patient-controlled analgesia
Under most circumstances, the suggested dose of morphine sulfate is 1 to 2 mg per patient administered bolus, with a lock-out interval of 6 to 10 minutes. Concurrent constant infusions are not generally recommended, but they may be helpful in patients with severe, continuous pain (eg, trauma).

Intrathecal administration (preservative-free formulation)
Administer 0.2 to 1 mg as a single injection, which may provide adequate pain relief for up to 24 hours.

Administration of more than 2 mg of the 0.5 mg/mL concentration or more than 1 mL of the 1 mg/mL concentration is not recommended. If pain is not relieved, consider other routes of administration. Repeated intrathecal dose not recommended.

Epidural administration (preservative-free formulation)
Typical administration of 5 mg in the lumbar spine region is recommended to provide adequate relief for up to 24 hours. If adequate pain relief does not occur in 1 hour, a dose of 1 to 2 mg, not to exceed 10 mg/24 hours can be given. Continuous infusion of 2 to 4 mg/24 hours (0.08 to 0.16 mg/hour) can also be used. The dose can be increased 1 to 2 mg/ day; doses of up to 30 mg/day have been used for severe pain.

These recommendations are the usual dosage ranges and may not be appropriate for all patients. Debilitated, elderly, or hepatically or renally impaired patients may require lower doses or prolonged dosage intervals.

Morphine sulfate is the preferred analgesic for critically ill patients. Hydromorphone may be used as an alternative. Fentanyl is the preferred agent in patients with hemodynamic instability, in patients experiencing histamine release with morphine, and in patients with morphine allergy. Meperidine is generally not recommended for use because the active metabolite normeperidine may accumulate and produce central nervous system stimulation. (See practice parameters for analgesia and sedation in suggested readings.)

In the management of cardiogenic pulmonary edema, morphine sulfate decreases anxiety and dilates pulmonary and systemic veins.

Dosage equivalents

fentanyl 0.1 mg = hydromorphone 1.5 mg = meperidine 100 mg = morphine 10 mg

If patients are switched to a different route or different opioid analgesic, it is recommended that they receive two thirds of the equianalgesic dose.

Dose or interval adjustment may be necessary in patients with renal insufficiency (creatinine clearance <50 mL/minute) or hepatic insufficiency.

Monitor

Pain relief, respiratory effects (use with caution in patients who are compromised or on concomitant respiratory depressants), central nervous system effects (sedation, euphoria, pupillary constriction), allergic reactions (some products contain sulfites), physical and psychological dependence, constipation (provide stool softeners as needed), urinary retention, and blood pressure (hypotension, especially with rapid infusion), nausea, vomiting, dizziness, and hypotension.

Tolerance develops with chronic use and coincides with the development of physical dependence, which can occur after only 2 weeks of therapy. Need to slowly taper dose over several days to minimize the effects. Signs of withdrawal include anxiety, tachycardia, and gastrointestinal distress.

Morphine releases histamine and therefore should be used with caution in patients with asthma.

In some patients (head trauma), the pattern and degree of pain are important diagnostic indicators. Examine all appropriate alternatives.

Protect from light: no (may darken upon prolonged exposure)

Special considerations

Use the preservative-free formulation for intrathecal and epidural administration.

pH: 2.5 to 6.5 (may be slightly variable depending on formulation)

Stability

Relative stability at pH $\leq$4; degradation increases at neutral or alkaline pH. Darkening of solution (darker than pale yellow) indicates degradation. Stable for at least 24 hours at room temperature.

Solution compatibility: D_5W, NS, $D_{10}W$, $\frac{1}{2}$NS, and LR

Compatible drugs

Allopurinol sodium
Amikacin sulfate
Aminophylline
Amiodarone HCl
Ampicillin sodium
Ampicillin sodium-
  sulbactam sodium
Amsacrine
Atenolol
Atracurium besylate
Aztreonam
Bumetanide
Calcium chloride
Cefazolin sodium
Ceftizoxime sodium
Cefoperazone sodium
Cefotaxime sodium
Cefotetan disodium
Cefoxitin sodium
Ceftazidime
Ceftriaxone sodium
Cefuroxime sodium

Chloramphenicol sodium
  succinate
Cisplatin
Clindamycin phosphate
Cyclophosphamide
Cytarabine
Dexamethasone sodium
  phosphate
Digoxin
Diltiazem HCl
Dopamine HCl
Doxorubicin HCl
Doxycycline hyclate
Enalaprilat
Erythromycin lactobionate
Esmolol HCl
Famotidine
Filgrastim
Fluconazole
Foscarnet sodium
Gentamicin sulfate
Heparin sodium

Hydrocortisone sodium
succinate
IL-2
Insulin, regular
Labetalol HCl
Lidocaine HCl
Magnesium sulfate
Melphalan HCl
Methotrexate sodium
Methyldopate HCl
Methylprednisolone sodium
succinate
Metoclopramide HCl
Metoprolol tartrate
Metronidazole
Mezlocillin sodium
Midazolam HCl
Moxalactam disodium
Nafcillin sodium
Nitroprusside sodium
Norepinephrine bitartrate
Ondansetron HCl
Oxacillin sodium

Oxytocin
Paclitaxel
Pancuronium bromide
Penicillin G potassium
Piperacillin sodium
Pipercillin sodium-
tazobaxam sodium
Potassium chloride
Propranolol HCl
Ranitidine HCl
Sodium bicarbonate
Teniposide
Ticarcillin disodium
Ticarcillin disodium-
clavulante potassium
Tobramycin sulfate
Trimethoprim-
sulfamethoxazole
Vancomycin HCl
Vecuronium bromide
Vinorelbine tartrate
Zidovudine

Incompatible drugs

Acyclovir sodium
Amphotericin B
Amrinone lactate
Azathioprine
Cefepime HCl
Folic acid
Furosemide
Ganciclovir sodium
Meperidine HCl

Methicillin sodium
Minocycline HCl
Pentamidine isethionate
Pentobarbital sodium
Phenobarbital sodium
Phenytoin sodium
Propofol
Sargramostim

NAFCILLIN SODIUM
Nafcil®, Apothecon, and other manufacturers

Methods of administration
Intramuscular (deep intragluteal injection), direct intravenous injection (dilute with 15 to 30 mL of NS and administer into a vein or into the tubing of a freely flowing compatible intravenous solution over 5 to 10 minutes), and intermittent intravenous infusion (over 10 to 15 minutes)

Dosing and administration
Standard: 500 to 1500 mg/50 mL and 2000 mg/100 mL of D_5W or NS

Nafcillin is a penicillinase-resistant penicillin that is active against most gram-positive and gram-negative aerobic cocci including penicillinase-producing and nonpenicillinase-producing strains of *Staphylococcus aureus, Staphylococcus epidermidis, and Staphylococcus saprophyticus*; groups A, B, C, and G streptococci; *Streptococcus pneumonia*e, and some viridans streptococci. Enterococci, including *Enterococcus, faecalis,* are usually resistant to nafcillin.

Treatment of osteomyelitis; septicemia; skin, soft-tissue, and CNS infections; and endocarditis
Administer 500 to 2000 mg every 4 to 6 hours.

No dosage reduction is necessary in patients with renal insufficiency. Minimal removal of medication by hemodialysis; no supplement required. Patients with concomitant renal and hepatic failure should have their dose reduced by as much as 50% of normal. Dosage adjustment recommended for patients with hepatic failure.

Monitor
Signs of infection (temperature, white blood cell count with differential), culture and susceptibility, hypersensitivity reactions, hematologic reactions (eg, neutropenia, which is immediately reversible on discontinuation of drug), phlebitis (eg, intravenous sites should be inspected and rotated fre-

quently), signs of central nervous system toxicity (neuromuscular hyperirritability and convulsions), and liver function.

Nafcillin is contraindicated for use in patients with a severe, documented allergy to penicillin antibiotics. It should be used cautiously in patients with allergies to cephalosporin (3% to 15% cross-reactivity), or carbapenem antibiotics (eg, imipenem), as cross-reactivity may exist.

Protect from light: no

Special considerations
If concomitant aminoglycoside use is needed, administer at least 1 hour from the nafcillin and flush tubing prior to administration.

pH: 6 to 8.5 (in D_5W)

Stability
Not stable at pH greater than 8 or below 5; when reconstituted, stable at room temperature for at least 24 hours, or for 4 days when refrigerated.

Solution compatibility: D_5W, NS, D_5NS, $D_{10}W$, and LR

Compatible drugs

Acyclovir sodium	Fluconazole
Atropine sulfate	Foscarnet sodium
Cyclophosphamide	Heparin sodium
Diazepam	Hydromorphone HCl
Enalaprilat	Magnesium sulfate
Esmolol HCl	Morphine sulfate
Famotidine	Perphenazine
Fentanyl citrate	Zidovudine

Incompatible drugs

Amphotericin B
Amrinone lactate
Ascorbic acid
Azathioprine sodium
Aztreonam sodium
Chloramphenicol sodium
    succinate
Cytarabine
Diltiazem HCl
Dobutamine HCl
Doxycycline hyclate
Droperidol
Folic acid
Haloperidol lactate
Hydralazine HCl
Hydrocortisone sodium
    succinate
Hydroxyzine HCl

Insulin, regular
Labetalol HCl
Meperidine HCl
Metaraminol bitartrate
Methicillin sodium
    succinate
Methylprednisolone
Minocycline HCl
Nalbuphine HCl
Pentamidine isethionate
Pentazocine lactate
Promazine HCl
Promethazine HCl
Protamine sulfate
Pyridoxine HCl
Quinidine gluconate
Verapamil HCl
Zidovudine

Methods of administration

Intramuscular, subcutaneous, direct intravenous injection, and continuous intravenous infusion

Dosing and administration

Standard: 0.4 mg/mL (undiluted if by direct IV injection); for continuous intravenous infusion, prepare 1 mg naloxone in 100 mL of D_5W or NS

Narcotic overdose (known or suspected)

An initial dose of 0.4 mg to 2 mg of naloxone may be administered by direct intravenous injection; this may be repeated at 2- to 3-minute intervals, as necessary. Additional doses may be necessary in 20 to 60 minutes. If no response is observed after 10 mg of naloxone have been administered, the diagnosis of narcotic-induced or partial narcotic-induced toxicity should be questioned. Reduces opioid-induced respiratory depression, central nervous system depression, and hypotension.

Continuous infusion: An intravenous loading dose of 0.4 mg followed by 0.1 to 0.4 mg/hour can be used. Infusion can be titrated by 0.2 mg/hour at 2- to 3-hour intervals. The amount of medication needed should be based on clinical response and continued until the opiate effects are no longer present.

Narcotic-induced sedation or respiratory depression

Administer 0.1 to 0.2 mg by direct intravenous injection every 2 to 3 minutes as needed. Typically does not require more than 0.6 mg. This dose should allow for reversal of somnolence while maintaining a reasonable amount of analgesia. In elderly patients, dilute a dose of 0.4 mg with 9 mL of D_5W or NS and give 2 mL of this solution to reverse respiratory depression by lessening the myocardial work load. Dose may need to be repeated every 15 to 30 minutes until the opioid effects are no longer present.

In the absence of an intravenous line access, naloxone can be administered sublingually or through the endotracheal route. Administer in a dose of 0.8 mg in 10 mL of NS in the endotracheal tube and repeat in 1 minute if necessary. No adjustment necessary for renal dysfunction.

Monitor
Reversal of effects (eg, narcotic toxicity), respiratory rate, heart rate, and blood pressure. Severe narcotic withdrawal may occur in individuals physically dependent on opiates.

Protect from light: yes

Special considerations: none

pH: 2.5 to 5 (may vary with product)

Stability
Unstable with alkaline solutions; most stable in the pH range of 2.5 to 5; stable at room temperature for at least 24 hours.

Solution compatibility: D_5W and NS

Compatible drugs

Limited data available (see general guidelines above)

Incompatible drugs

Propofol

NITROGLYCERIN
Nitro-Bid®, Hoechst Marion Roussel, and other manufacturers

Methods of administration
Direct intravenous injection and continuous intravenous infusion

Dosing and administration
Standard: 100 mg/500 mL (200 µg/mL) of D_5W; concentrated, 100 mg/250 mL in a deep line (400 µg/mL)

Unstable angina, congestive heart failure, pulmonary edema, severe hypertension
May initiate with a direct intravenous injection of 12.5 to 25 µg or a continuous infusion at a dose of 5 to 20 µg/minute and increase by 10 µg/minute at 3- to 5-minute intervals. Usual maximum is 400 µg/minute. Rarely, a patient may require 500 µg/minute.

Infarct size and complications may be reduced with nitroglycerin (best if given within 4 hours).

Monitor
Blood pressure (hypotension), relief of angina, heart rate (eg, reflex tachycardia), nausea, vomiting, lightheadedness, flushing, headache, and dizziness. Sustained infusions (greater than 48 hours) may result in tachyphylaxis or tolerance. May elevate or worsen intracranial pressure in patients with reduced intracranial compliance. Rarely, methemoglobinemia may occur; it can be reversed with methylene blue.

Protect from light: no

Special considerations
Use of filters should be avoided; rate control device recommended for continuous infusion; administer in glass container, or in McGaw IV bags (will adsorb to some PVC bags).

pH: 3 to 6.5

Stability

Stable in weakly acidic solutions at pH 3 to 5; store at room temperature.

Solution compatibility: D_5W, NS, LR, D_5NS, and $^1/_2NS$

Compatible drugs

Amiodarone HCl
Amrinone lactate
Atracurium besylate
Diltiazem HCl
Dobutamine HCl
Dopamine HCl
Esmolol HCl
Famotidine
Fluconazole
Haloperidol lactate
Heparin sodium

Insulin, regular
Labetalol HCl
Lidocaine HCl
Midazolam Hcl
Nitroprusside sodium
Pancuronium bromide
Ranitidine HCl
Streptokinase
Tacrolimus
Vecuronium bromide

Incompatible drugs

Alteplase
Phenytoin sodium
Propofol

NITROPRUSSIDE SODIUM
Nitropress®, Abbott Laboratories, and other manufacturers

Method of administration
Continuous intravenous infusion (do not give by direct intravenous injection)

Dosing and administration
Standard: 50 mg/250 mL of D_5W (200 µg/mL) concentrated, 100 mg/250 mL

Hypertensive crisis, afterload reduction postmyocardial infarction, or in severe left ventricular dysfunction
Initiate with 0.1 µg/kg/minute by continuous intravenous infusion and titrate dose in increments of 0.5 µg/kg/minute every 5 to 10 minutes until desired blood pressure is achieved. Most patients respond at 0.75 to 3 µg/kg/minute to a maximum of 10 µg/kg/minute.

Monitor
Blood pressure (eg, hypotension), dizziness, headache, diaphoresis, thiocyanate and cyanide toxicity, nausea, and vomiting.

Thiocyanate and cyanide toxicity: Nitroprusside is metabolized by the liver to cyanide, which is then metabolized to thiocyanate. Thiocyanate is then eventually eliminated by the kidneys.

Cyanide toxicity: hypotension, nausea, vomiting, palpitations, bradycardia, hyperpnea, agitation, agitation followed by combative behavior, convulsions, dilated pupils, coma, and death. Sodium thiosulfate may be added to nitroprusside infusions at a ratio of 10:1 to help prevent cyanide toxicity.

Thiocyanate toxicity: muscular fatigue, abdominal pain, nausea, vomiting, confusion, tinnitus, convulsions, coma, and death. Risk factors for development of thiocyanate toxicity include hepatic dysfunction, serum C_N>2.0 mg/dL and administration of less than 2 µg/kg/minute for at least 48 hours.

Hydroxocobalamin (25 mg/hour) may be administered

concurrently for those risk factors for developing thiocyanate toxicity. Dialysis may also help remove thiocyanate. Thiocyanate levels may not be readily available to be clinically useful.

Protect from light: yes

Special considerations:
Infusion device is recommended for continuous infusions.

pH: 3.5 to 6 in D_5W

Stability
Do not use if discolored (straw, brownish pink, light orange, brown). A blue color indicates degradation and breakdown to cyanide.

Compatible drugs

Amrinone lactate	Insulin, regular
Atracurium besylate	Labetalol HCl
Diltiazem HCl	Lidocaine HCl
Dobutamine HCl	Midazolam HCl
Dopamine HCl	Morphine sulfate
Enalaprilat	Nitroglycerin
Esmolol HCl	Pancuronium bromide
Famotidine	Tacrolimus
Heparin sodium	Vecuronium bromide

Incompatible drugs

Amphotericin B	Haloperidol
Ascorbic acid	Hydralazine HCl
Azathioprine sodium	Hydroxyzine HCl
Ceftazidime (sodium bicarbonate)	Imipenem-cilastatin sodium
Chlorpromazine HCl	Pentazocine lactate
Diphenhydramine HCl	Prochlorperazine edisylate
Promethazine HCl	Propofol
Erythromycin lactobionate	Quinidine gluconate

NOREPINEPHRINE BITARTRATE
Levophed®, Sanofi Winthrop Pharmaceuticals

Method of administration
Continuous intravenous infusion

Dosing and administration
Standard: 8 mg/250 mL of D_5W (32 µg/mL); concentrated, 16 mg/250 mL (64 µg/mL)

Hypotension associated with low systemic vascular resistance
Initiate at 0.1 µg/kg/minute and increase by 0.1 µg/kg/minute every 5 to 10 minutes up to 3 µg/kg/minute based on hemodynamic response.

Stop norepinephrine infusion slowly over 6 to 24 hours to avoid abrupt hypotension.

norepinephrine bitartrate 2 mg = norepinephrine base 1 mg

Monitor
Cardiac index (especially in patients with poor ventricular function), blood pressure, serum creatinine (renal dysfunction, especially in septic patients), heart rate (bradycardia), arrhythmias (especially in volume-depleted patients), and allergy (some products may contain sulfites).

Extravasation may cause tissue necrosis and sloughing (administer into large vein). Phentolamine can be administered for extravasations (5 to 10 mg in 10 to 15 mL of NS and inject into area).

Protect from light: yes (undiluted)

Special considerations
Infusion device is recommended. Administration should occur through a central line if possible. Otherwise, norepinephrine should be administered through an antecubital vein of the arm, although a femoral vein may also be used.

pH: 3 to 4.5

Stability
Stable at pH 3.6 to 6 in D_5W; do not use if brown discoloration; stable in solution for at least 24 hours at room temperature if pH is 5.6.

Solution compatibility: D_5NS and D_5W (preferred)

Compatible drugs

Amiodarone HCl	Labetalol HCl
Amrinone	Meropenem
Diltiazem HCl	Midazolam
Dopamine HCl	Morphine sulfate
Famotidine	Potassium chloride
Haloperidol lactate	
Heparin sodium	
Hydrocortisone sodium succinate	

Incompatible drugs

Aminophylline	Insulin, human
Amphotericin B	Lidocaine HCl
Azathioprine sodium	Pentobarbital sodium
Folic acid	Phenobarbital sodium
Furosemide	Sodium bicarbonate
Ganciclovir sodium	

OFLOXACIN INJECTION
Floxin®, McNeil Pharmaceutical

Method of administration
Intermittent intravenous infusion (over 60 minutes); *not* for intramuscular or subcutaneous injection

Dosing and administration
Standard: 200 mg/50 mL or 400 mg/100 mL of D_5W or NS

Ofloxacin is a quinolone antibiotic that has a spectrum of activity similar to that of ciprofloxacin. The activity of ofloxacin against susceptible gram-positive organisms is approximately equal to that of ciprofloxacin. The activity of ofloxacin against susceptible gram-negative bacteria is slightly less than that of ciprofloxacin.

Treatment of skin and skin structure, urinary tract, upper and lower respiratory tract infections, and sexually transmitted diseases
Administer 200 to 400 mg every 12 hours. Typically used for 7 to 10 days.

Ofloxacin is contraindicated for use in patients with severe, documented allergy to quinolone antibiotics.

In patients with a creatinine clearance of 10 to 30 mL/minute, administer 100% of dose every 12 to 24 hours. For a creatinine clearance less than 10 mL/minute, increase the dosing interval to every 24 hours. Does not require dose or interval adjustment with hepatic insufficiency. A negligible amount of ofloxacin is removed by hemodialysis.

Monitor
Signs of infection (temperature, white blood cell count with differential), culture and susceptibility, gastrointestinal effects (nausea, diarrhea, abdominal pain), central nervous system effects (drowsiness, headache, and insomnia), and toxicity (neuromuscular hyperirritability and convulsions), and hypersensitivity reactions.

Ofloxacin has been shown to increase serum theophylline and cyclosporine concentrations and increase the effects of warfarin.

Protect from light: yes (concentrate and premix solutions in bottles)

Special considerations: none

pH: 3.5 to 5.5 (in concentrate for injection); 3.8 to 5.8 (in D_5W)

Stability
Solution is light yellow to amber in color; stable for 72 hours at room temperature.

Solution compatibility: D_5NS, D_5W and NS

Compatible drugs

Ampicillin sodium

Incompatible drugs

Cefepime HCl

PANCURONIUM BROMIDE
Pavulon®, Organon Inc., and other manufacturers

Methods of administration
Direct intravenous injection (over 15 to 90 seconds), and intermittent intravenous infusion, continuous intravenous infusion

Dosing and administration
Standard: 50 mg/250 mL of D_5W or NS (concentrated solution of 100 mg/250 mL)

Immobilization for mechanical ventilation

Pancuronium is an intermediate-acting, nondepolarizing, neuromuscular blocking agent (onset of effect: 3 to 5 minutes; duration: 60 to 90 minutes, depending on dose). Initiate therapy with a dose of 0.07 to 0.1 mg/kg (4 to 10 mg) by direct intravenous injection over 15 to 30 seconds. As a maintenance dose, administer 0.03 to 0.04 mg/kg (2 to 4 mg) by direct intravenous injection every 3 hours. Dosage interval can be increased as needed every 2 hours, then titrate by 0.015 to 0.02 mg/kg (1 to 2 mg) every 2 to 4 hours (maximum of 0.06 mg/kg every hour). As an alternative, a continuous infusion can be used at a rate of 0.02 to 0.04 mg/kg/hour to a maximum of 0.6 mg/kg/hour.

Note: The infusion rate recommendations are mg/kg/hour (not μg/kg/minute) as is the case with most of the other neuromuscular blocking agents.

Pancuronium is the preferred neuromuscular blocker for most critically ill patients. Vecuronium is preferred for those patients with cardiac disease or hemodynamic instability in whom tachycardia may be deleterious. (See practice parameters for sustained neuromuscular blockade in the suggested readings.)

Indications for neuromuscular blocking agents in the intensive care unit include endotracheal intubation, status epilepticus, status asthmaticus, adult respiratory distress syndrome, neuromuscular toxins, tetanus, and hypothermia.

DO NOT PARALYZE PATIENT WITHOUT ADEQUATE SEDATION. Need to coadminister with medications that provide sedation, analgesia, or amnesia. Use precaution with pressure points on the eyes or skin, and provide prophylaxis for thrombosis.

Pancuronium is primarily excreted in the urine and should be used with caution in patients with renal disease. Half-life and serum concentrations are significantly increased in patients with renal insufficiency; therefore, doses should be decreased. Administer 50% of the dose in patients with a creatinine clearance of 10 to 50 mL/minute.

Monitor
Neuromuscular blockade (peripheral nerve stimulation with train-of-four monitoring every 4 to 8 hours with a goal of 2 to 4 twitches), hypertension and tachycardia, and convulsions (rare and usually in patients with predisposing factors such as head trauma).

Several risk factors place a patient at increased risk of prolongation of neuromuscular blockade: accumulation of drug or metabolite, electrolyte imbalance (hypokalemia, hypomagnesemia, and hypocalcemia), and medications including calcium channel blockers, corticosteroids, antiarrhythmics (eg, procainamide and quinidine), antibiotics (eg, aminoglycosides), and immunosuppressants. Chronic use of phenytoin or carbamazepine may result in resistance to neuromuscular blockade.

Pancuronium does not produce histamine-release hypotension, but provides modest to marked tachycardia and hypertension primarily from a vagolytic effect on the sinus node and blocking the re-uptake of norepinephrine. Use caution in patients who are cardiovascularly compromised; administration can lead to myocardial ischemia.

Protect from light: no

Special considerations: rate control device required

pH: 4

Stability
Stable for up to 24 hours at room temperature after dilution.

Solution compatibility: D_5W, NS, D_5NS, and LR

Compatible drugs

Aminophylline	Hydrocortisone sodium
Cefazolin sodium	succinate
Cefuroxime sodium	Isoproterenol
Cimetidine HCl	Lorazepam
Dobutamine HCl	Midazolam HCl
Dopamine HCl	Morphine sulfate
Epinephrine HCl	Nitroglycerin
Esmolol HCl	Nitroprusside sodium
Fentanyl citrate	Ranitidine HCl
Fluconazole	Trimethoprim-
Gentamicin sulfate	sulfamethoxazole
Heparin sodium	Vancomycin

Incompatible drugs

Diazepam
Pentobarbital
Phenobarbital
Propofol

PENICILLIN G POTASSIUM
Pfizerpen®, Pfizer Inc, and other manufacturers
PENICILLIN G SODIUM
Apothecon

Methods of administration
Intramuscular (deep in the upper outer quadrant of the buttocks), intermittent intravenous infusion (over 1 to 2 hours), intrathecal, and intra-articular

Dosing and administration
Standard: 1 million U/50 mL of NS, 2 to 3 million U/100 mL of NS

Penicillin G is a natural penicillin that is active against many gram-positive aerobic cocci including nonpenicillinase-producing *Staphylococcus aureus* and *Staphylococcus epidermidis*; *Streptococcus pneumoniae*; groups A, B, C, G, H, K, L or M streptococci; viridans streptococci; nonenterococcal group D streptococci; and some strains of enterococci.

Penicillin G is also active against some gram-negative aerobic bacteria (nonpenicillinase-producing strains), eg, *Neisseria meningitidis, Neisseria gonorrhoeae, Haemophilus influenzae, Haemophilus parainfluenzae, Bordetella pertussis,* and *Eikenella corrodens.* It is also active against some anaerobic bacteria, including *Actinomyces israelii, Clostridium tetani, Clostridium perfringens,* and *Clostridium botulinum,* Eubacteria, *Peptostreptococcus* sp, *Propionibacterium* sp and some spirochetes (*Treponema pallidum, Borrelia burgdorferi*).

Treatment of respiratory tract, endocarditis, and central nervous system infections
Administer 2 to 24 million U daily in divided doses every 4 to 6 hours. Typical dose is 2 million U every 4 hours. Higher doses necessary for central nervous system infections.

1 million U of penicillin potassium contain
1.7 mEq of potassium

Dosage adjustment recommended in patients with renal insufficiency. In patients with a creatinine clearance of 10 to 50 mL/minute, administer 75% of the dose every 4 hours. For a creatinine clearance less than 10 mL/minute, administer 20% to 50% of the dose every 4 hours. Dosage adjustment recommended in patients with hepatic failure when accompanied by renal failure.

Monitor
Signs of infection (temperature, white blood cell count with differential), culture and susceptibility, potassium (penicillin G potassium), hypersensitivity reactions, and signs of central nervous system toxicity (neuromuscular hyperirritability and convulsions).

Penicillin G potassium is contraindicated in patients with severe, documented allergy to penicillin antibiotics. It should be used cautiously in patients with allergies to cephalosporin or carbapenem antibiotics, as cross-reactivity may exist. Cross-reactivity occurs in 3% to 15% of patients.

Protect from light: no

Special considerations
If concomitant aminoglycoside use is needed, administer at least 1 hour from the penicillin and flush tubing prior to administration.

pH: 6.0 to 8.5 (reconstituted solution) penicillin potassium
6 to 7.5 (reconstituted solution) penicillin sodium

Stability
Unstable at pH of 5.5 and below and above 8.5; stable for 24 hours at room temperature and for 7 days with refrigeration.

Solution compatibility: D_5W and NS

Compatible drugs (penicillin G potassium)

Acyclovir sodium
Amiodarone HCl
Cyclophosphamide
Diltiazem HCl
Enalaprilat
Esmolol HCl
Fluconazole
Foscarnet sodium
Heparin sodium
Hydromorphone HCl
Labetalol HCl
Magnesium sulfate
Meperidine HCl
Morphine sulfate
Perphenazine
Potassium chloride
Tacrolimus
Verapamil HCl

Incompatible drugs (penicillin G potassium)

Aminophylline
Amphotericin B
Amrinone lactate
Ascorbic acid
Chlorpromazine HCl
Dobutamine HCl
Dopamine HCl
Doxycycline hyclate
Erythromycin lactobionate
Ganciclovir sodium
Haloperidol lactate
Hydroxyzine HCl
Labetalol HCl
Minocycline HCl
Pentamidine isethionate
Pentazocine lactate
Pentobarbital sodium
Phenytoin sodium
Prochlorperazine edisylate
Promazine HCl
Promethazine HCl
Protamine sulfate
Quinidine gluconate

Compatible drugs (penicillin G sodium)

Meperidine HCl

Incompatible drugs (penicillin G sodium)

Aminophylline
Amphotericin B
Amrinone lactate
Chlorpromazine HCl
Cytarabine
Dobutamine HCl
Doxycycline hyclate
Erythromycin lactobionate
Ganciclovir sodium
Haloperidol lactate
Hydroxyzine HCl
Labetalol HCl
Metaraminol bitartrate
Methylprednisolone sodium
    succinate
Minocycline HCl

Papaverine HCl
Pentamidine isethionate
Pentazocine lactate
Pentobarbital sodium
Phenobarbital sodium

Phentolamine mesylate
Prochlorperazine edisylate
Promethazine HCl
Protamine sulfate
Quinidine gluconate

PENTOBARBITAL SODIUM
Nembutal®, Abbott Laboratories, and other manufacturers

Methods of administration
Intramuscular (deep), direct intravenous injection (undiluted), and continuous intravenous infusion

Dosing and administration
Standard: 2500 mg/50 mL of D_5W or NS

Increased intracranial pressure or status epilepticus (induction of coma for treatment unresponsive to other therapy)
Initiate therapy at 5 to 10 mg/kg over 1 to 2 hours. Maintenance infusions are typically administered at a rate of 1 mg/kg/hour, up to 2 mg/kg/hour. Do not exceed a rate of administration of 50 mg/minute.

Pentobarbital is used to manage increases in intracranial pressure and cerebral ischemia, but is not the drug of choice for any seizure disorder. In patients refractory to conventional anticonvulsants, pentobarbital may be used to control status epilepticus.

No dosage or interval adjustments required in patients with renal insufficiency. Reduce dose with severe liver dysfunction.

Monitor
Desired effects (resolution of seizures), decreased intracranial pressure, central nervous system effects (drowsiness, and confusion), respirations, cardiovascular effects (arrhythmias), EEG, blood pressure (hypotension), tolerance or psychological and physical dependence with prolonged use, and serum pentobarbital concentrations.

Pharmacokinetic considerations

Sample collection:

Obtain 2 to 3 hours after loading dose or

Obtain 12 and 24 hours after maintenance infusion begins

Therapeutic range:

20 to 40 µg/mL (therapeutic coma)

1 to 5 µg/mL (hypnotic effects)

Protect from light: no

Special considerations

Intra-arterial administration has resulted in arterial spasm and gangrene that has required intervention.

pH: 9 to 10.5

Stability

Low pH may cause precipitation; do not use if precipitate forms.

Solution compatibility: D_5W (<8 g/L), $D_{10}W$, LR, NS (<8 g/L), and D_5NS

Compatible drugs

Acyclovir sodium
Insulin, regular

Incompatible drugs

Amikacin sulfate
Ampicillin sodium
Amrinone lactate
Ascorbic acid
Atracurium besylate
Aztreonam
Benzquinamide HCl
Benztropine mesylate
Buprenorphine HCl
Butorphanol tartrate
Cefamandole nafate
Cefazolin sodium
Cefmetazole sodium
Cefonicid sodium
Cefotaxime sodium
Cefotetan disodium

Cefoxitin sodium
Ceftazidime (L-arginine)
Ceftizoxime
Ceftriaxone sodium
Cefuroxime
Chlorpromazine HCl
Cimetidine HCl
Clindamycin phosphate
Codeine phosphate
Cyclosporine
Diphenhydramine HCl
Dobutamine HCl
Doxycycline hyclate
Droperidol
Ephedrine HCl
Epinephrine HCl
Erythromycin lactobionate
Esmolol HCl
Fentanyl citrate
Gentamicin sulfate
Haloperidol lactate
Hyaluronidase
Hydralazine HCl
Hydrocortisone sodium
     succinate
Hydromorphone HCl
Hydroxyzine HCl
Isoproterenol HCl
Ketorolac (D_5W)

Lidocaine HCl
Meperidine HCl
Methadone HCl
Midazolam HCl
Minocycline HCl
Morphine sulfate
Moxalactam (D_5W)
Nalbuphine HCl
Norepinephrine bitartrate
Ondansetron HCl
Pancuronium bromide
Papaverine
Penicillin G potassium
Penicillin G sodium
Pentamidine isethionate
Pentazocine lactate
Perphenazine
Phenotolamine mesylate
Phenytoin sodium
Prochlorperazine
Promazine HCl
Promethazine HCl
Propofol
Protamine sulfate
Pyridoxine HCl
Quinidine gluconate
Ranitidine HCl
Tobramycin sulfate
Verapamil HCl

PHENOBARBITAL
various manufacturers

Methods of administration
Intramuscular (deep), and direct intravenous injection (over 5 minutes or 60 mg/minute)

Dosing and administration
Standard: 130 mg/mL (direct IV injection)

Prophylactic management and treatment of tonic-clonic seizures
Administer 3 to 6 mg/kg by direct intravenous injection over 5 minutes (50 mg/minute). Repeat every 20 minutes until seizures are controlled or a cumulative dose of 20 mg/kg (1.5 g maximum). Begin maintenance 12 hours after load. Then administer 3 to 6 mg/kg/day by direct intravenous injection or orally in divided doses every 8 to 12 hours for a maximum of 120 mg every 8 hours. Subsequent doses should be based on serum drug levels.

Administer 15 to 20 mg/kg as a loading infusion for status epilepticus. Dilute in 100 to 150 mL D_5W or NS and infuse at 50 mg/minute.

If patient is maintained on phenobarbital, administer 4 mg/kg of phenobarbital intravenous injection for every 5 mg/L increase in phenobarbital serum level desired.

Phenobarbital can lower intracranial pressure due to suppression of cerebral metabolism and cerebral blood flow. The drug has no anxiolytic or analgesic effects.

Similar to phenytoin in onset and degree of effectiveness; however, there is an increase in risk of side effects with phenobarbital including sedation and respiratory depression. Has also been used to lower serum bilirubin or serum lipid concentration in the management of chronic cholestasis.

Monitor
Resolution of seizures, sedation, respiratory depression, ECG (cardiovascular depression, especially at high doses), blood pressure (hypotension, especially in patients with pre-existing

cardiovascular disease, hypovolemia, and the elderly). Extravasation of phenobarbital may cause tissue damage secondary to the alkaline pH of the drug. Following chronic administration, the drug must be withdrawn slowly to avoid the possibility of precipitating withdrawal in a patient who is physically dependent.

Drug interactions with valproic acid, carbamazepine, and warfarin.

Pharmacologic considerations
Sample collection:
Obtain trough within 60 minutes prior to dose
Therapeutic range:
10 to 40 µg/mL

Protect from light: no

Special considerations: none

pH: approximately 9.2 to 10.2

Stability: unstable in an acidic medium

Solution compatibility: D_5W, NS, $D_{10}W$, LR, and ½NS

Compatible drugs

Enalaprilat
Sufentanil citrate

Incompatible drugs

Ampicillin sodium	Cefuroxime sodium
Amrinone lactate	Cimetidine HCl
Atracurium besylate	Chlorpromazine HCl
Buprenorphine HCl	Clindamycin phosphate
Cefmetazole sodium	Codeine phosphate
Cefotaxime sodium	Cyclosporine
Cefotetan disodium	Diphenhydramine HCl
Cefoxitin sodium	Dobutamine HCl

Doxycycline hyclate
Droperidol
Ephedrine sulfate
Epinephrine HCl
Erythromycin lactobionate
Esmolol HCl
Haloperidol lactate
Hydralazine HCl
Hydrocortisone sodium
    succinate
Hydromorphone HCl
Hydroxyzine HCl
Imipenem-cilastatin sodium
Isoproterenol HCl
Levophanol bitartrate
Lidocaine HCl
Meperidine HCl
Methadone HCl
Midazolam HCl
Minocycline HCl
Morphine sulfate
Norepinephrine bitartrate

Ondansetron HCl
Pancuronium bromide
Penicillin G potassium/
    sodium
Pentamidine isethionate
Pentazocine lactate
Phenytoin sodium
Prochlorperazine mesylate
Promazine HCl
Promethazine HCl
Propofol
Protamine sulfate
Pyridoxine HCl
Quinidine gluconate
Ranitidine HCl
Sodium bicarbonate
Streptomycin sulfate
Succinylcholine chloride
Tetracycline HCl
Thiamine HCl
Vancomycin HCl
Verapamil HCl

PHENYLEPHRINE HYDROCHLORIDE
Neo-Synephrine® HCl, Sanofi Winthrop Pharmaceuticals

Methods of administration
Direct intravenous injection (mix 1 mL [1 mg/mL] of phenylephrine HCl with 9 mL sterile water), and continuous intravenous infusion

Dosing and administration
Standard: 10 mg/250 mL of D_5W (0.04 mg/mL); concentrated, 100 mg/500 mL

Hypotensive shock
Initiate at a dose of 25 to 40 µg/minute as a continuous intravenous infusion. Titrate by increments of 25 to 50 µg/minute every 10 to 20 minutes. Patients usually require a maintenance dose of 40 to 60 µg/minute.

Empirically reserved for hypotension associated with low systemic vascular resistance refractory to volume expansion and inotropic support. Phenylephrine is a useful alternative in patients who develop unacceptable tachycardia and tachydysrhythmias with dopamine or norepinephrine.

Monitor
Blood pressure, heart rate (eg, bradycardia), angina, cardiac output, urine output, IV infiltration (causes tissue necrosis and sloughing), and allergic reactions (may contain sulfites), and excessive peripheral vasoconstriction.

Phentolamine can be used for extravasation. Mix 5 mg with 9 mL of NS and inject into extravasated area.

Protect from light: no

Special considerations: rate control device recommended

pH: 3 to 6.5

Stability

Stable over pH range of 3.5 to 7.5; do not use if a precipitate forms (eg, brown); not stable with alkalis, ferric salts, and other metals.

Solution compatibility: D_5W, NS, LR, $D_{10}W$, and 1/2NS

Compatible drugs

Amiodarone HCl	Famotidine
Amrinone lactate	Haloperidol lactate
Etomidate	Zidovudine

Incompatible drugs

Amphotericin B	Minocycline HCl
Azathioprine sodium	Pentamidine isethionate
Ganciclovir sodium	Propofol
Insulin, human	

PHENYTOIN SODIUM
various manufacturers

Methods of administration

Intermittent intravenous infusion, direct intravenous injection, intramuscular (generally not recommended because of erratic absorption and pain at injection site), and *not* subcutaneous (because of the potential for tissue damage)

Dosing and administration

Standard: Dose/100 mL of NS (dilution not generally recommended because of the risk of phenytoin precipitation; however, there are several published reports of routine usage)

Tonic-clonic seizures (grand mal), simple partial, and complex partial, and prevention of seizures posttrauma

A loading dose of 18 to 20 mg/kg (actual body weight) (750 µg/kg/minute for pediatric patients) should be administered slowly intravenously, at a rate not exceeding 50 mg/minute (this will require approximately 20 minutes in a 70-kg patient). Patients should be on a monitor with cardiac rate and blood pressure display when receiving 300 mg or more per dose. Patients with advanced age, those who are debilitated, and patients with unstable cardiovascular status may require administration at a slower rate of 10 to 20 mg/minute. Propylene glycol solvent increases risk of cardiovascular problems. The loading dose should be followed by maintenance doses of 4 to 6 mg/kg/day intravenously, divided into 8- to 12-hour intervals.

Flush the IV line with 5 cc NS before administering phenytoin to decrease the risk of precipitation. Following intravenous administration, NS should be administered in the catheter to decrease irritation. If a patient has subtherapeutic drug blood levels, 3.5 mg/kg of phenytoin can be given for every 5 mg/L increase desired in patient's serum phenytoin concentration.

(desired level − actual level) × 0.7 (Vd) × weight in kg
Vd=Volume of distribution.

In patients with end-stage renal failure or other reasons to have decreased albumin, dose should be based on unbound phenytoin level or adjusted phenytoin concentrations (use equation shown in box below).

Note: Assure patency of IV before and after administration of phenytoin. A CVP line is preferred but not mandatory: Peripheral IVs should be inserted in a large arm vein with a 20 G bore minimum. Phenytoin can cause severe tissue extravasation* when infiltrated into subcutaneous tissue. Peripheral IVs should be inserted in a large vein as proximal as possible. Hand or foot vein access should be avoided whenever possible. Check site frequently for extravasation. Rapid treatment of extravasation can decrease the severity of tissue damage. Recommended treatment as follows: 1) stop infusion, 2) withdraw fluid subcutaneously at the IV site, 3) infiltrate the subcutaneous tissue around the affected area with hydrocortisone 100 mg, 4) document in patient's record, 5) complete incident report, 6) complete adverse drug reaction report.

Therapeutic drug monitoring considerations
(It is important to assess whether the patient is at steady state in interpreting the levels.)

Sample collection:
Obtain trough within 60 minutes prior to dose
Therapeutic range:
Total: 10 to 20 µg/mL
Unbound: 1 to 2 µg/mL

Phenytoin serum level can be corrected to reflect increased free drug in patients with renal dysfunction or decreased albumin in the following manner:

$$C\ calc = \frac{C\ OBS}{(0.25)\ albumin + 0.1}$$

For elderly and trauma patients, see Anderson GD, et al. Revised Winter-Tozer equation. *Ann Pharmacother.* 1997;31:279.

This equation is useful to assist with the decision whether to obtain an unbound level. Adjustments of dose should be made based on measured unbound concentrations.

Monitor
Seizure occurrence (motor manifestations or electrographic seizures), phenytoin blood levels, blood pressure (hypotension, may be rate related), cardiovascular effects (increased risk with hemodynamic instability, elderly, compromised pulmonary function, and co-existing cardiac arrhythmias), skin necrosis at intravenous site, heart rate (eg, bradycardia, may be rate related), albumin, drug concentration-related effects such as nystagmus, blurred vision, drowsiness, and hyperglycemia.

Many medications interact with phenytoin to cause both lowering and raising of serum concentrations. All concomittant medications should be evaluated for potential interactions and reassessed with the elimination or addition of any medication.

Protect from light: no

Special considerations
Intermittent infusions should be administered with in-line 0.22 micron filter because of the potential of precipitation of drug. The risk of soft-tissue injury can be minimized by using a large vein for infusion, followed by normal saline and avoid giving in hand or foot veins.

pH: 10 to 12.3

Stability
Not stable in medications diluted in D_5W (stability is concentration dependent); use only if solution is clear; drug may precipitate at a pH <11.5; use immediately, stable for only 4 hours.

Solution compatibility: NS

*reaction may not appear until hours to days (see description of "Purple Glove Syndrome")

Compatible drugs

Esmolol HCl
Famotidine
Fluconazole

Foscarnet sodium
Tacrolimus

Incompatible drugs

Amikacin sulfate
Aminophylline
Bretylium tosylate
Chloramphenicol
Ciprofloxacin
Clindamycin phosphate
Codeine phosphate
Diltiazem
Diphenhydramine
Dobutamine HCl
Enalaprilat
Gentamicin sulfate
Heparin sodium
Hydromorphone HCl
Hydroxyzine HCl
Insulin, regular
Levorphanol bitartrate

Lidocaine HCl
Meperidine HCl
Methadone HCl
Morphine sulfate
Nitroglycerin
Penicillin G potassium
Pentobarbital sodium
Phenobarbital sodium
Phytonadione
Potassium chloride
Procainamide HCl
Promazine HCl
Promethazine HCl
Propofol
Secobarbital sodium
Vancomycin HCl sodium
    succinate

PHOSPHATE
potassium or sodium
various manufacturers

Method of administration
Intermittent intravenous infusion (infused over 4 to 6 hours)

Dosing and administration
Standard: Dose/100 to 500 mL of D_5W or NS over no less than 4 hours

Hypophosphatemia
For mild (serum phosphorous concentration 1.5 to 1.9 mg %), moderate (1.0 to 1.4 mg %), and severe hypophosphatemia (<1.0 mg %), administer 0.125 mmol/kg, 0.25 mmol/kg, and 0.3 mmol/kg phosphorous, respectively. Administer over 4 to 6 hours by intermittent intravenous infusion. Subsequent doses should be based on serum phosphate levels and patient response. Serum sodium and potassium concentrations should help dictate selection of product. Typically requires 24 to 36 hours of therapy because of the need to replenish intracellular stores of phosphate.

Identify and eliminate the causes of hypophosphatemia, including impaired intestinal absorption and increases in renal excretion. Hypokalemia and hypomagnesemia may induce hypophosphatemia; may need to replace these two electrolytes concurrently with phosphate supplementation.

Sodium phosphate	=	3 mmol phosphate/mL and 4.0 mEq sodium/mL
Potassium phosphate	=	3 mmol phosphate/mL and 4.4 mEq potassium/mL

Typically expressed as mmols of phosphate instead of mEq to help avoid confusion:

1 mmol phosphate	=	31 mg phosphorus
1 mg phosphorus	=	0.032 mmol

Replace phosphate cautiously in patients with renal insufficiency or end-stage renal disease.

Monitor
Signs of deficiency including neuromuscular effects (muscle weakness, hypoflexia, paresthesias), respiratory failure, congestive heart failure, central nervous system effects (confusion, seizures and coma), tremors, gastrointestinal effects (diarrhea, nausea, stomach pain). Hemolysis, platelet dysfunction, and metabolic acidosis rarely occur.

Other monitoring parameters: serum phosphate level (take 1 hour after administration of phosphate), electrolytes (hypercalcemia may precipitate or aggravate hypophosphatemia), sodium, and renal status (use caution in patients with dysfunction).

Avoid hyperphosphatemia, which may cause hypocalcemia, renal failure, hypotension, and death.

Protect from light: no

Special considerations: infusion device recommended

pH: 7 to 7.8 potassium phosphate

Stability
Phosphate salts may precipitate with calcium salts; stable at room temperature for 24 hours.

Solution compatibility: D_5W, NS, $D_{10}W$, and $^1/_2NS$ (potassium)

Compatible drugs (potassium phosphate)

Ciprofloxacin	Esmolol HCl
Diltiazem HCl	Famotidine
Enalaprilat	Labetalol HCl

Incompatible drugs (potassium phosphate)

Dobutamine HCl

Compatible drugs (sodium phosphate)

Ciprofloxacin

Incompatible drugs (sodium phosphate)

Calcium chloride
Calcium gluconate

PIPERACILLIN SODIUM STERILE
Pipracil®, Lederle Laboratories

Methods of administration
Intramuscular (maximum of 2 g into the upper outer area of the buttocks), direct intravenous injection (administer into a vein or into the tubing of a freely flowing compatible intravenous solution over 3 to 5 minutes), and intermittent intravenous infusion (over 20 to 30 minutes)

Dosing and administration
Standard: 4 g/50 mL of NS or D_5W

Piperacillin is an extended-spectrum penicillin that is active against most gram-positive and gram-negative aerobic cocci (except penicillinase-producing strains), some gram-positive aerobic and anaerobic bacilli, and many gram-negative anaerobic bacilli. The drug is also active against many gram-negative aerobic bacilli, including the Enterobacteriaceae and *Pseudomonas* sp. Piperacillin is generally more active in vitro on a weight basis against the Enterobacteriaceae and *Pseudomonas aeruginosa* than the other extended-spectrum penicillins.

For treatment of the following serious infections: septicemia, nosocomial pneumonia, intra-abdominal, aerobic and anaerobic gynecologic, and skin and soft-tissue
Administer 12 to 18 g daily in divided doses every 4 to 6 hours.

Complicated urinary tract infections
Administer 8 to 16 g intravenously daily (125 to 200 mg/kg/dose) in divided doses every 6 to 8 hours.

General
Dosage adjustment is required for patients with renal insufficiency (less than 30 mL/minute). For patients with a creatinine clearance of 10 to 30 mL/minute, administer every 6 to 8

hours. For a creatinine clearance less than 10 mL minute, increase the interval to every 8 to 12 hours. For patients receiving hemodialysis, administer 1g after hemodialysis, then 2 g every 8 hours. Limited data are available for dosage adjustments in patients with hepatic failure.

Monitor
Signs of infection (temperature, white blood cell count with differential), culture and susceptibility, hypersensitivity reactions, signs of bleeding, and signs of central nervous system toxicity (neuromuscular hyperirritability and convulsions).

Piperacillin is contraindicated for use in patients with severe, documented allergy to penicillin antibiotics. Piperacillin should be used cautiously in patients with allergies to cephalosporin or carbapenem antibiotics, as cross-reactivity may exist. Cross-reactivity with cephalosporins occurs in 3% to 15 % of patients.

Protect from light: no

Special considerations
If concomitant aminoglycoside use is needed, administer at least 1 hour from the piperacillin sodium and flush tubing prior to administration.

pH: 5.5 to 7.5.

Stability
Stable over pH range of 4.5 to 8.5; stable for at least 24 hours at room temperature or for 7 days with refrigeration.

Solution compatibility: D_5W, NS, D_5NS, and LR

Compatible drugs

Acyclovir sodium
Allopurinol sodium
Aztreonam
Ciprofloxacin
Cyclophosphamide
Diltiazem HCl
Enalaprilat
Esmolol HCl
Famotidine
Fludarabine phosphate
Foscarnet sodium
Heparin sodium
Hydromorphone HCl

IL-2
Labetalol HCl
Magnesium sulfate
Melphalan HCl
Meperidine HCl
Morphine sulfate
Perphenazine
Ranitidine HCl
Tacrolimus
Teniposide
Verapamil HCl
Zidovudine

Incompatible drugs

Amphotericin B
Amrinone lactate
Azathioprine sodium
Chlorpromazine HCl
Dobutamine HCl
Doxycycline hyclate
Filgrastim
Fluconazole
Ganciclovir sodium
Haloperidol lactate
Hydroxyzine HCl

Minocycline HCl
Nalbuphine HCl
Ondansetron HCl
Papaverine HCl
Pentamidine isethionate
Pentazocine lactate
Promethazine HCl
Protamine sulfate
Quinidine gluconate
Sargramostim
Vinorelbine tartrate

PIPERACILLIN SODIUM STERILE-TAZOBACTAM SODIUM
Zosyn®, Lederle Laboratories

Methods of administration

Intermittent intravenous infusion (over 20 to 30 minutes), intramuscular (maximum of 2 g into the upper outer area of the buttocks), and direct intravenous injection (administer into a vein or into the tubing of a freely flowing compatible intravenous solution over 3 to 5 minutes)

Preparation and administration

Standard: 3.375 g/50 mL of D_5W or NS

Piperacillin sodium-tazobactam sodium is an extended-spectrum penicillin plus a β-lactamase inhibitor that has a wide spectrum of activity and is active against many gram-positive and gram-negative aerobic and anaerobic bacteria. Because tazobactam has a high affinity for and binds to certain β-lactamases that generally inactivate piperacillin, concurrent administration of the drugs results in a synergistic bactericidal effect that expands the spectrum of activity of piperacillin against many β-lactamase-producing organisms that are resistant to piperacillin alone, including piperacillin-resistant strains of *Staphylococcus* sp, *Haemophilus* sp, Enterobacteriaceae, and *Bacteroides* sp. Tazobactam generally acts as an irreversible inhibitor and inactivates both plasmid and chromosome-mediated β-lactamases. *Pseudomonas*-resistant organisms are generally also resistant to piperacillin sodium and tazobactam sodium combination.

Lower respiratory tract, urinary tract, skin and skin structure, gynecological, bone and joint infections, and septicemia caused by susceptible organisms
Given 3.375 g every 6 hours.

3.375 grams of combined drug = 3 g piperacillin and 0.375 g tazobactam

Dosage adjustment required for patients with renal insufficiency (creatinine clearance less than 30 mL/minute). For patients with a creatinine clearance of 10 to 30 mL/minute, increase the interval to every 6 to 8 hours. For a creatinine clearance less than 10 mL/minute, administer every 8 to 12 hours. In patients with hemodialysis, administer 750 mg after dialysis, then 2.25 g every 8 hours. Limited data are available for dosage adjustments in patients with hepatic failure.

Monitor
Signs of infection (temperature, white blood cell count with differential), culture and susceptibility, hypersensitivity reactions, platelet count (thrombocytopenia), and central nervous system toxicity (neuromuscular hyperirritability and convulsions).

Piperacillin is contraindicated for use in patients with severe, documented allergy to penicillin antibiotics. It should be used cautiously in patients with allergies to cephalosporin or carbapenem antibiotics, as cross-reactivity may exist. Cross-reactivity with cephalosporins occurs in 3% to 15% of patients.

Protect from light: no

Special considerations
If concomitant aminoglycoside use is needed, administer at least 1 hour from the piperacillin sodium-tazobactam sodium and flush tubing prior to administration.

pH: 4.5 to 6.8

Stability
In compatible diluent, the solution is stable for 24 hours at room temperature or for 7 days with refrigeration.

Solution compatibility: D_5W, NS, and *not* LR

Compatible drugs

Aminophylline
Aztreonam
Bumetanide
Buprenorphine HCl
Butorphanol tartrate
Calcium gluconate
Carboplatin
Carmustine
Cefepime HCl
Cimetidine HCl
Clindamycin phosphate
Cyclophosphamide
Cytarabine
Dexamethasone sodium
    phosphate
Diphenhydramine HCl
Dopamine HCl
Enalaprilat
Etoposide
Fluconazole
Fludarabine phosphate
Fluorouracil
Furosemide
Heparin sodium
Hydrocortisone sodium
    phosphate
Hydrocortisone sodium
    succinate
Hydromorphone HCl
Ifosfamide
Leucovorin calcium
Lorazepam
Magnesium sulfate
Mannitol
Meperidine HCl
Mesna
Methotrexate sodium
Methylprednisolone
    sodium succinate
Metoclopramide HCl
Metronidazole
Morphine sulfate
Ondansetron HCl
Plicamycin
Potassium chloride
Ranitidine HCl
Sargramostim
Sodium bicarbonate
Thiotepa
Trimethoprim-
    sulfamethoxazole
Vinblastine sulfate
Vincristine sulfate
Zidovudine

Incompatible drugs

Acyclovir sodium
Amphotericin B
Chlorpromazine HCl
Cisplatin
Dacarbazine
Daunorubicin HCl
Dobutamine HCl
Doxorubicin HCl
Doxycycline hyclate
Droperidol
Famotidine
Ganciclovir sodium

Haloperidol lactate
Hydroxyzine HCl
Idarubicin HCl
Miconazole
Minocycline HCl
Mitomycin

Mitoxantrone HCl
Nalbuphine HCl
Prochlorperazine edisylate
Promethazine HCl
Vancomycin HCl

POTASSIUM CHLORIDE
various manufacturers

Methods of administration
Intermittent intravenous infusion, continuous intravenous infusion, do not give by direct intravenous injection or retrograde infusion

Dosing and administration
Standard: Maximum dose 20 mEq/100 mL of D_5W or NS for peripheral IV or 40 mEq/100 mL for central line

Hypokalemia
Administer 20 to 40 mEq potassium chloride by intermittent intravenous infusion and repeat dose based on serum potassium concentrations and clinical symptoms. Mild and moderate deficiency may require administration on a 24- and 4-hour basis, respectively. Severe depletion may require successive doses or a continuous infusion until the potassium rises to 3 mEq/L and the patient is asymptomatic.

Potassium chloride should not be administered at a rate faster than 10 mEq/hour in a nonintensive care unit area. In an intensive care unit, potassium chloride can be administered at 40 mEq/hour if given via a central line with an infusion device.

Identify and eliminate causes of hypokalemia, if possible, including concomitant medications (eg, amphotericin B, diuretics, β-agonists, and aminoglycosides). Hypokalemia is generally refractory to potassium administration if hypomagnesemia coexists. Administer potassium cautiously in patients with renal insufficiency.

Monitor
Clinical signs of hypokalemia: muscle weakness, fatigue, paresthesias, cramps, respiratory depression, and hypoactive reflexes.

An ECG is advised for infusion of severely depleted patients or those receiving more than 20 mEq/hour.

Other monitoring parameters: serum potassium concentrations (obtain at least 1 hour after the end of the potassium infusion), acid/base status (a 0.1 unit increase in arterial pH inversely decreases the serum potassium concentration by 0.6 mEq/L), fluid status (input and output), ECG changes (eg, hypokalemia: paroxysmal tachycardia), magnesium (may result in inadequate response if hypomagnesemia exists), renal status (decreases elimination of potassium), pain and irritation upon infusion (consider central administration if available), and extravasation (administer hyaluronidase 150 units/mL into the infiltration site to decrease damage).

Monitor for signs of hyperkalemia including prolonged PR interval with AV block and widened QRS interval. Calcium gluconate is useful for treatment of hyperkalemia and peaked T waves.

Protect from light: no

Special considerations
An infusion device is recommended.

pH: 4 to 8

Stability
Admixtures stable for at least 24 hours at room temperature.

Solution compatibility: D_5W, NS, $D_{10}W$, 1/2NS, and LR

Compatible drugs

Acyclovir sodium	Chlordiazepoxide HCl
Allopurinol sodium	Chlorpromazine HCl
Aminophylline	Ciprofloxacin
Amiodarone HCl	Cyanocobalamin
Ampicillin sodium	Dexamethasone sodium
Atropine sulfate	phosphate
Aztreonam	Digoxin
Betamethasone sodium	Diltiazem HCl
phosphate	Diphenhydramine HCl
Calcium gluconate	Dobutamine HC

Dopamine HCl
Droperidol
Edrophonium chloride
Enalaprilat
Epinephrine HCl
Esmolol HCl
Estrogens, conjugated
Ethacrynate sodium
Famotidine
Fentanyl citrate
Filgrastim
Fludarabine phosphate
Fluorouracil
Furosemide
Heparin sodium
Hydralazine HCl
Idarubicin HCl
Insulin, regular
Isoproterenol HCl
Labetalol HCl
Lidocaine HCl
Magnesium sulfate
Melphalan HCl
Meperidine HCl
Methicillin sodium
Methoxamine HCl

Minocycline HCl
Morphine sulfate
Norepinephrine bitartrate
Ondansetron HCl
Oxacillin sodium
Oxytocin
Paclitaxel
Penicillin G potassium
Pentazocine lactate
Phytonadione
Piperacillin sodium-
    tazobactam sodium
Prednisolone sodium
    phosphate
Procainamide HCl
Prochlorperazine edisylate
Propranolol HCl
Sargramostim
Sodium bicarbonate
Succinylcholine chloride
Tacrolimus
Teniposide
Trimethobenzamide HCl
Vinorelbine tartrate
Zidovudine

Incompatible drugs

Amphotericin B
Amrinone lactate
Diazepam
Ergotamine tartrate
Erythromycin lactobionate
Haloperidol lactate

Mannitol
Methylprednisolone sodium
    succinate
Pentamidine isethionate
Phenytoin sodium

PROCAINAMIDE HYDROCHLORIDE
Pronestyl®, Apothecon, and other manufacturers

Methods of administration
Intramuscular, intermittent intravenous infusion, and continuous intravenous infusion

Dosing and administration
Standard: 2 g/500 mL of NS (4 mg/mL); maximum concentration of 4 g/500 mL

Treatment of atrial arrhythmias (including atrial fibrillation, atrial flutter, paroxysmal atrial tachycardia, and paroxysmal AV junctional rhythm), and ventricular arrhythmias including ventricular tachycardia, and PVCs not responsive to lidocaine
Administer an intravenous infusion of 50 to 100 mg at a rate not more than 20 to 30 mg/minute. Repeat until the arrhythmia is controlled. Alternatively, administer 12 to 17 mg/kg (typically 1000 mg) infused over 45 to 60 minutes. Maintenance infusion (once ventricular tachycardia is terminated) is generally 1 to 4 mg/minute.

Monitor
ECG, blood pressure (hypotension, consider slowing infusion rate if blood pressure drops 15 mm Hg), widening of QRS complex and prolongation of QT interval (consider slowing infusion rate if less than 50%), ventricular tachycardia, AV nodal block, or other arrhythmias.

Therapeutic drug monitoring considerations
> Sample collection:
>> Obtain trough within 30 minutes prior to dose
> Therapeutic range:
>> Procainamide: 4 to 10 µg/mL
>> NAPA: 15 to 25 µg/mL
>> Procainamide + NAPA: 10 to 30 µg/mL

Procainamide is metabolized in the liver to NAPA, which has some class IC antiarrhythmic activity. Procainamide is 50% renally eliminated and 50% hepatically eliminated. NAPA is more than 90% renally eliminated.

Protect from light: no

Special considerations: none

pH: 4 to 6

Stability

May be stored at room temperature; admixture stable at room temperature for 24 hours; solutions darker than amber should be discarded; procainamide may be subject to greater decomposition in D_5W unless the admixture is refrigerated or pH adjusted.

Solution compatibility: D_5W, NS (preferred), D_5NS, and ½NS

Compatible drugs

Amiodarone HCl
Amrinone lactate
Azathioprine sodium
Cefamandole nafate
Chloramphenicol sodium
   succinate
Diltiazem HCl
Ethacrynate sodium
Famotidine
Ganciclovir sodium
Heparin sodium
Hydralazine HCl
Hydrocortisone sodium
   succinate
Imipenem-cilastatin sodium
Metronidazole HCl
Minocycline HCl
Potassium chloride
Ranitidine HCl

Incompatible drugs

Bretylium tosylate
Ceftizoxime
Esmolol HCl
Milrinone
Phenytoin sodium

PROPOFOL
Diprivan® 1% Injectable emulsion, Zeneca Pharmaceuticals

Method of administration
Continuous intravenous infusion (undiluted)

Dosing and administration
Ready to use oil-in-water emulsion that contains soybean oil, glycerol, and egg lecithin (10 mg/mL concentration); available in 50 and 100 mL vials

Agitation/sedation (eg, patients maintained on ventilator)
Propofol has sedative, hypnotic, anxiolytic, and anterograde amnestic effects. Because of the rapid onset of action (1 to 2 minutes) and short-acting effects (10 to 15 minutes), the drug is administered only by continuous intravenous infusion. In most patients the initial infusion is 5 µg/kg/minute and titrated in increments of 5 µg/kg/minute every 10 minutes.

Typical maintenance infusion is 5 to 50 µg/kg/minute. Evaluate level of sedation and assess central nervous system function daily throughout maintenance to determine the minimum dose of propofol required for sedation. When discontinuing propofol, be sure to taper dose 5 µg/kg/minute every 15 minutes to avoid abrupt arousal.

Midazolam and propofol are the preferred agents for short-term treatment of anxiety only in the critically ill patient. (See practice parameters for intravenous analgesia and sedation in the suggested readings.) Propofol may be used in combination with benzodiazepines (midazolam) or opiates (morphine).

The use of propofol in patients with head injury is associated with either unchanged or slightly decreased intracranial pressure.

Shake prior to administration. Should be administered without dilution directly from the vial. With prolonged infusion, the intravenous tubing must be changed every 12 hours.

Propofol is a caloric source = 10% intralipid (1.1 kcal/mL)

The presence of cirrhosis or renal dysfunction does not significantly affect the pharmacokinetics of propofol.

Monitor
Sedation, ECG (reports of asystole, heart block and other types of arrhythmias), blood pressure (infusion-rate dependent hypotension; bolus doses not recommended because of significant hypotension), infection, heart rate (bradycardia), triglycerides (long-term use, more than 4 days, has been associated with an increase in triglycerides), respiratory acidosis (most commonly during weaning patient from ventilator; seen in 10% of patients), patients with egg allergies should not receive this.

Infection caused by a variety of organisms has been associated with the failure to use aseptic technique in the preparation and administration of propofol.

Patients who are elderly, debilitated, cardiovascularly compromised (ejection fraction <50%), hypovolemic, and on concomitant β-adrenergic antagonists are at greatest risk of hypotension.

Protect from light: no

Special considerations
Aseptic technique must be maintained because of risk for bacterial growth. Do not use filters with a pore size less than 5 μm. Needs to be administered via a central line. Contains 0.005% disodium edetate to retard the growth of microorganisms, in the event of accidental extrinsic contamination.

pH: 7 to 8.5

Stability: do not use if separation of emulsion occurs

Solution compatibility

D$_5$W (dilution should not be less than 2 mg/mL); not recommended to dilute, but if used, mix in D$_5$W at a concentration *not less than* 2 mg/mL.

Compatible drugs

Limited data available

Incompatible drugs

Alfentanil HCl
Amikacin sulfate
Aminophylline
Amphotericin B
Ampicillin sodium
Ampicillin sodium-
    sulbactam sodium
Amrinone lactate
Atracurium besylate
Atropine sulfate
Bretylium tosylate
Calcium chloride
Calcium gluconate
Cefazolin sodium
Cefotetan disodium
Cefoxitin sodium
Ceftazidime
Ceftizoxime sodium
Cimetidine HCl
Ciprofloxacin
Cisatracurium
Cisplatin
Clindamycin phosphate
Cyclophosphamide
Dexamethasone sodium
    phosphate
Diazepam
Digoxin

Diphenhydramine HCl
Dobutamine HCl
Dopamine HCl
Doxorubicin
Droperidol
Ephedrine sulfate
Epinephrine
Esmolol HCl
Famotidine
Fluconazole
Gentamicin sulfate
Heparin sodium
Hydralazine HCl
Hydrocortisone sodium
    succinate
Imipenem disodium/
    cilastatin sodium
Labetolol
Lidocaine HCl
Lorazepam
Meperidine HCl
Methylprednisolone sodium
    succinate
Metoclopramide
Mezlocillin sodium
Midazolam HCl
Morphine sulfate
Naloxone HCl

Nitroglycerin
Nitroprusside sodium
Pancuronium bromide
Pentobarbital sodium
Phenobarbital sodium
Phenylephrine HCl
Phenytoin
Potassium chloride
Propranolol HCl
Ranitidine HCl
Sodium bicarbonate
Succinylcholine chloride
Sufentanil citrate
Ticarcillin disodium-
    clavulanate potassium
Tobramycin sulfate
Vancomycin HCl
Vecuronium bromide
Verapamil HCl

PROTAMINE SULFATE
various manufacturers

Method of administration
Direct intravenous injection (administer 50 mg over 10 minutes)

Dosing and administration
Typically given by direct intravenous injection

Heparin sodium overdose
Amount of drug administered is based on heparin dose: 1 mg protamine sulfate neutralizes 90 USP units of heparin activity derived from bovine lung tissue and 115 USP units of heparin derived from porcine intestinal mucosa to a maximum dose of 50 mg in 10 minutes.

In concentration, give 10 mg/mL over 1 to 3 minutes. If 30 to 60 minutes have elapsed since heparin sodium has been given, then 0.75 mg protamine for each 100 units of heparin should be administered. If heparin was administered as a continuous intravenous infusion, 50 mg of protamine can be administered after the infusion has stopped. If heparin was given subcutanously, use 1 to 1.5 mg protamine per 90 units heparin sodium. Administer 50 mg initially, then give the remainder over 8 to 16 hours.

Heparin rebound has occurred rarely after 8 to 18 hours of protamine administration and has been associated with anticoagulation and bleeding.

Monitor
Signs of bleeding, allergic reactions (in patients with an allergy to fish and in patients sensitized to protamine, such as diabetic patients receiving protamine-insulin preparations), blood pressure (hypotension with too rapid an infusion), and aPTT.

Protect from light: no

Special considerations: none

pH: 6 to 7 (injection); 6.5 to 7.5 (reconstitution with sterile water)

Stability
Stable for greater than 24 hours at room temperature.

Solution compatibility: D_5W, NS

Compatible drugs

Limited data available

Incompatible drugs

Amphotericin B
Ampicillin sodium
Ampicillin sodium-
   sulbactam sodium
Cefamandole nafate
Cefazolin sodium
Cefmetazole sodium
Cefonicid sodium
Cefoperazone sodium
Cefotaxime sodium
Cefotetan disodium
Cefoxitin sodium
Ceftizoxime sodium
Ceftriaxone sodium
Cefuroxime sodium
Chloramphenicol sodium
   succinate
Dexamethasone sodium
   phosphate
Folic acid
Furosemide
Heparin sodium

Hydrocortisone sodium
   succinate
Insulin (human)
Ketorolac tromethamine
Methicillin sodium
Methylprednisolone sodium
   succinate
Mezlocillin sodium
Moxalactam disodium
Nafcillin sodium
Oxacillin sodium
Penicillin G potassium
Penicillin G sodium
Pentamidine isethionate
Pentobarbital sodium
Phenobarbital sodium
Piperacillin
Streptokinase
Ticarcillin disodium
Ticarcillin disodium-
   clavulanate potassium

RANITIDINE HYDROCHLORIDE
Zantac®, Glaxo Wellcome Inc.

Methods of administration

Intramuscular (undiluted), direct intravenous injection (should be diluted in 20 mL of NS or D_5W and administered over at least 5 minutes), intermittent intravenous infusion, and continuous intravenous infusion

Dosing and administration

Standard: 50 mg/100 mL of D_5W or NS (minimum of 20 mL) or 150 mg/250 mL of D_5W or NS

Gastrointestinal disorders

Administer 50 mg by intermittent intravenous infusion over 15 to 20 minutes or direct intravenous injection every 6 to 8 hours (not to exceed 400 mg/day). For a continuous infusion, administer 6.25 mg/hour (150 mg ranitidine/day) and titrate to maintain a gastric pH > 4 for prophylaxis or pH >7 for treatment. For patients requiring a more rapid elevation of gastric pH, the continuous infusion may be preceded by a 50-mg loading dose administered by intermittent intravenous infusion. Doses up to 2.5 mg/kg/hour have been used in patients with hypersecretory conditions.

Ranitidine has been used for prevention of stress ulceration, treatment of gastric or duodenal ulcers, and control of gastric pH in critically ill patients.

Dose or interval adjustment needed in patients with renal insufficiency (creatinine clearance <50 mL/minute); administer 50 mg intravenously every 24 hours. In patients receiving hemodialysis, administer 50 mg ranitidine daily.

Monitor

Symptomatic response to therapy, gastric pH, signs of bleeding (eg, occult blood), central nervous system effects (dizziness, headache, confusion; mental status changes occur most often in elderly patients, or in patients with renal or hepatic dysfunction; less frequently than with cimetidine), hematologic effects (neutropenia, thrombocytopenia), and serum creatinine (monitor renal status to correct dose).

Protect from light: no

Special considerations: none

pH: 6.7 to 7.3

Stability
Slight darkening does not affect potency; stable for at least 24 hours at room temperature when mixed with diluent.

Solution compatibility: D_5W, NS, $D_5^1/_2NS$, and $D_{10}W$

Compatible drugs

Acyclovir sodium	Fluconazole
Allopurinol sodium	Foscarnet sodium
Aminophylline	Heparin sodium
Amsacrine	Labetalol HCl
Atracurium besylate	Melphalan HCl
Aztreonam	Meperidine HCl
Bretylium tosylate	Meropenem
Cefepime	Methotrexate sodium
Cefmetazole	Morphine sulfate
Ceftazidime	Nitroglycerin
Ciprofloxacin	Ondansetron HCl
Cisplatin	Paclitaxel
Cyclophosphamide	Pancuronium bromide
Cytarabine	Piperacillin sodium
Diltiazem HCl	Piperacillin sodium-
Dobutamine HCl	tazobactam sodium
Dopamine HCl	Procainamide HCl
Enalaprilat	Sargramostim
Esmolol HCl	Tacrolimus
Filgrastim	Vecuronium bromide
Fludarabine phosphate	Zidovudine

Incompatible drugs

Amphotericin B
Cefamandole nafate
Cefoxitin sodium
Cefuroxime sodium
Diazepam
Hetastarch

Hydroxyzine HCl
Midazolam HCl
Pentobarbital sodium
Phenobarbital sodium
Phytonadione
Propofol

RIFAMPIN
various manufacturers

Method of administration
Intermittent intravenous infusion, and *not* intramuscular or subcutaneous

Dosage and administration
Standard: 600 mg in 100 mL D_5W (over 30 minutes)

Rifampin has activity against *Legionella pneumophila, Mycobacterium avium-intracellulare, Mycobacterium tuberculosis*, as well as methicillin-resistant *Staphylococcus aureus* and methicillin-resistant *Staphylococcus epidermidis*.

Treatment of active tuberculosis
Rifampin should only be used in combination with other agents because of a high rate of resistance. Administer 10 mg/kg (up to 600 mg) by intermittent intravenous infusion over 30 minutes twice weekly.

Synergy for Staphylococcus aureus *infections*
Administer 300 to 600 mg twice daily by intermittent intravenous infusion over 30 minutes. Used in combination with other antibiotics.

Adjustment of dose is necessary in patients with hepatic impairment.

Monitor
Signs of infection (temperature, white blood cell count and differential); culture and susceptibility; serum creatinine; blood urea nitrogen; fluid status; complete blood count; may discolor urine, tears, sweat red-orange (contact lenses may be permanently stained); signs of liver dysfunction (AST, ALT, persistent flu-like symptoms, nausea, vomiting).

May decrease plasma concentrations of digoxin, cyclosporine, oral anticoagulants, theophylline, barbiturates, and quinidine.

Protect from light: yes (intact vials protected from excessive light)

Special considerations: none

Stability
Constituted solution stable for 24 hours at room temperature. Manufacturers recommend that the time for preparation and administration not exceed 4 hours because of the potential for precipitation.

Solution compatibility: D_5W (preferable) and NS

Compatible drugs

Limited data available

Incompatible drugs

Diltiazem HCl
Minocycline HCl

ROCURONIUM BROMIDE
Zemuron™, Organon Inc.

Methods of administration
Direct intravenous injection and continuous intravenous infusion

Dosing and administration
Standard: 200 mg/100 mL of D_5W or NS

Immobilization for mechanical ventilation

Rocuronium is an intermediate-acting nondepolarizing neuromuscular blocker with rapid onset of action (onset of effect: 1 minute; duration: 30 to 40 minutes, depending on dose). When administered in larger doses, it has an onset similar to succinylcholine, and therefore may be considered an alternative to succinylcholine when a rapid onset of blockade is needed. In contrast to succinylcholine, rocuronium has a duration similar to other intermediate-acting neuromuscular blockers.

Initiate blockade with a dose of 0.6 mg/kg by direct intravenous injection. Then administer 4 to 15 µg/kg/minute as a maintenance infusion in patients monitored by peripheral nerve stimulation. The manufacturer recommends that obese patients receive rocuronium based on actual body weight.

Indications for neuromuscular blocking agents in the intensive care unit include endotracheal intubation, sedation, status epilepticus, status asthmaticus, adult respiratory distress syndrome, neuromuscular toxins, tetanus, and hypothermia.

DO NOT PARALYZE PATIENT WITHOUT ADEQUATE SEDATION. Need to coadminister with medications that provide sedation, analgesia, or amnesia. Use precaution with pressure points on the eyes or skin, and provide prophylaxis for thrombosis.

In patients with renal failure, the clinical duration is similar to that in patients with normal function. Adjust dose or interval in patients with hepatic insufficiency. Clinical duration is approximately 1.5 times that in patients with normal hepatic function. The elderly may also experience an increased duration of blockade.

Monitor

Neuromuscular blockade (peripheral nerve stimulation with train-of-four monitoring every 4 to 8 hours with a goal of 2 to 4 twitches), blood pressure (hypotension), heart rate (tachycardia or bradycardia), and convulsions (rare and usually in patients with predisposing factors such as head trauma).

Several risk factors place a patient at increased risk of prolongation of neuromuscular blockade: accumulation of drug or metabolite, electrolyte imbalance (hypokalemia, hypomagnesemia, and hypocalcemia), and medications including calcium channel blockers, corticosteroids, antiarrhythmics (eg, procainamide and quinidine), antibiotics (eg, aminoglycosides), and immunosuppressants. Chronic use of phenytoin or carbamazepine may result in resistance to neuromuscular blockade.

No histamine-release hypotension (or secondary to ganglionic block); however, there is some vagal-block tachycardia at higher doses.

Protect from light: no

Special considerations: rate control device required

pH: 4

Stability: use within 24 hours once diluted

Solution compatibility: D_5W, NS, and LR

Drug compatibility

Limited data available

SODIUM BICARBONATE
various manufacturers

Methods of administration
Direct intravenous injection, intermittent intravenous infusion, and continuous intravenous infusion

Dosing and administration
Standard: 50 mEq/100 mL of D_5W; 100 mEq/1000 mL of D_5W

Respiratory or metabolic acidosis
Can be administered during cardiopulmonary resuscitation in a dose of 1 mEq/kg as a direct intravenous injection; repeat with a dose of 0.5 mEq/kg every 10 minutes as needed. If ABGs are available, dose should be based on patient's base deficit:

$$NaHCO_3 \text{ dose (mEq)} = 0.5 \text{ (L/kg)} \times \text{body weight (kg)}$$
$$\times \text{ desired increase in serum bicarbonate}$$

To treat metabolic acidosis, a 7.5% to 8.4% solution may be infused over 10 minutes. In patients with persistent acidosis, continuous infusion of 0.15 to 0.4 mEq/kg/hour may be used. Titrate in increments of 0.1 to 0.25 mEq/kg/hour to a maximum of 1.25 mEq/kg/hour.

Sodium bicarbonate should be used only after adequate alveolar ventilation has been established and effective cardiac compressions are provided.

Tricyclic antidepressant overdose
Sodium bicarbonate is the drug of choice to reverse QRS and QT widening and seizures caused by tricyclic overdose. It is indicated if QRS >0.16 msec.

Monitor
Arterial pH (goal: 7.10 to 7.20), serum bicarbonate concentration (goal greater than 10 mEq/L), potassium (hypokalemia), sodium (hypernatremia), fluid status (input and output), and ECG. Administration of a loop diuretic (eg, furosemide) may

minimize risk of hypernatremia and volume overload. Fluid overload may result in hypoxia (monitor arterial blood gas). Bicarbonate administration may result in overalkalinization and a paradoxical transient acidosis.

Protect from light: no

Special considerations: none

pH: 7 to 8.5

Stability
Do not use if solution unclear or contains a precipitate; do not mix with acid labile solutions; stored at room temperature.

Solution compatibility: D_5W, NS, D_5NS, $D_{10}W$, and 1/2NS

Compatible drugs

Acyclovir sodium	Granisetron HCl
Asparaginase	Heparin sodium
Aztreonam	Ifosfamide
Cefepime HCl	Insulin, regular
Ceftriaxone sodium	Melphalan HCl
Cyclophosphamide	Methylprednisolone sodium
Cytarabine	succinate
Daunorubicin HCl	Morphine sulfate
Dexamethasone sodium	Paclitaxel
phosphate	Piperacillin sodium-
Doxorubicin HCl	tazobactam sodium
Etoposide	Potassium chloride
Famotidine	Teniposide
Filgrastim	Vancomycin HCl
Fludarabine phosphate	

Incompatible drugs

Amiodarone HCl	Amrinone lactate
Amphotericin B	Ascorbic acid
Ampicillin sodium	Azathioprine sodium

Buprenorphine HCl
Butorphanol tartrate
Calcium chloride
Calcium gluconate
Carboplatin
Carmustine
Cefmetazole sodium
Cefotaxime sodium
Cefotetan disodium
Cefoxitin
Cefuroxime sodium
Chlorpromazine HCl
Cisplatin
Codeine phosphate
Diazepam
Diltiazem
Diphenhydramine HCl
Dobutamine HCl
Dopamine HCl
Doxycycline hyclate
Epinephrine HCl
Ganciclovir sodium
Haloperidol lactate
Hydromorphone HCl
Hydroxyzine HCl
Idarubicin HCl
Imipenem-cilastatin sodium

Isoproterenol HCl
Labetalol HCl
Leucovorin calcium
Levorphanol bitartrate
Magnesium sulfate
Meperidine HCl
Methadone HCl
Metoclopramide HCl
Midazolam HCl
Minocycline HCl
Nalbuphine HCl
Norepinephrine bitartrate
Ondansetron HCl
Oxacillin sodium
Pentamidine isethionate
Pentazocine lactate
Pentobarbital sodium
Procaine HCl
Prochlorperazine edisylate
Promethazine HCl
Propofol
Quinidine gluconate
Sargramostim
Secobarbital sodium
Succinylcholine chloride
Thiamine HCl
Verapamil HCl

STREPTOKINASE
Streptase®, Astra USA, Inc., and other manufacturers

Methods of administration
Continuous intravenous infusion, intermittent intravenous infusion, and intra-arterial or intracoronary injection

Dosing and administration
Standard: 1,500,000 IU/150 mL of D_5W

Acute evolving transmural myocardial infarction
Administer streptokinase as soon as possible after onset of symptoms. Administer 1,500,000 IU within 60 minutes by intermittent intravenous infusion or 20,000 IU in 20 mL NS by direct intracoronary injection over 1 minute in the cardiac catheter laboratory, followed by 2000 IU per minute for 60 minutes (total dose 140,000 IU). The greatest benefit in mortality reduction was observed when streptokinase was administered within 4 hours, but statistically significant benefit has been reported up to 24 hours.

Pulmonary embolism, deep-vein thrombosis, arterial thrombosis, or embolism
Streptokinase treatment should be instituted as soon as possible after onset of the thrombotic event, preferably within 7 days. Administer a loading dose of 250,000 IU over 30 minutes, then 100,000 IU for 24 to 72 hours, depending on anatomic location (pulmonary 24 hours; deep-vein thrombosis 72 hours; and arterial thrombosis or embolism 24 to 72 hours).

Arteriovenous cannula occlusion
Before using streptokinase, an attempt should be made to clear the cannula by careful syringe technique, using heparinized saline solution. If this is unsuccessful, instill 250,000 IU streptokinase in 2 mL of solution into each occluded limb of the cannula over 25 to 35 minutes. Clamp off cannula limb(s) for 2 hours, aspirate, and then flush with NS.

General

Streptokinase is not indicated for management of ischemic stroke (see guidelines for thrombolytic therapy for acute stroke in suggested readings).

Monitor

Indication of reperfusion: documented by coronary angiography (infarct artery open), reduction of ST segment elevation, resolution of chest pain, elevation of total creatine kinase and MB-CK isoenzyme, and echocardiography (improvement in regional wall motion).

Other monitoring parameters: bleeding (eg, external bleeding around venipuncture sites, hypotension, hematuria, abdominal pain, headache, blurred vision), heart rate, extravasation (causes ecchymosis or inflammation) and aPTT.

Repeat doses of streptokinase may increase the risk of allergic reactions. Major allergic reactions are rare with the first dose. Neutralizing antibodies have been found with repeated administration, but the clinical relevance of this is unclear.

Protect from light: no

Special considerations

Rate control device recommended. Infuse intravenous solution using an in-line filter $\geq$ 0.45 micron.

pH: depends on diluent, but most stable at pH of 6 to 8

Stability

Most stable at pH of 6 to 8. Reconstituted solutions should be stored in the refrigerator. Manufacturers recommend that the drug be used within 8 hours of reconstitution.

Solution compatibility: NS (preferred), D_5W

Compatible drugs

Dobutamine HCl
Dopamine HCl
Heparin sodium

Lidocaine HCl
Nitroglycerin

Incompatible drugs

Azathioprine sodium
Chlorpromazine HCl
Ganciclovir sodium
Hydroxyzine HCl
Metaraminol (NS)
Minocycline HCl

Nalbuphine HCl
Pentamidine isethionate
Prochlorperazine edisylate
Promethazine HCl
Vancomycin HCl

TICARCILLIN DISODIUM
Ticar®, SmithKline Beecham Pharmaceuticals

Methods of administration
Intramuscular (do not exceed 2 g), direct intravenous injection (administer into a vein or into the tubing of a freely flowing compatible intravenous solution, not to exceed concentrations of 50 mg/mL), and intermittent intravenous infusion (over 20 to 30 minutes)

Dosing and administration
Standard: 1 to 4 g/50 mL of D_5W or NS

Ticarcillin disodium is an extended-spectrum penicillin that is active against most gram-positive and gram-negative aerobic cocci (except penicillinase-producing strains), some gram-positive aerobic and anaerobic bacilli, and many gram-negative anaerobic bacilli. The drug is also active against many gram-negative aerobic bacilli, including the Enterobacteriaceae and *Pseudomonas* sp. Piperacillin is generally more active in vitro on a weight basis than ticarcillin against the Enterobacteriaceae and *Pseudomonas aeruginosa*.

Treatment of septicemia, respiratory tract, skin and soft-tissue, and intra-abdominal infections, and infections of the female pelvis and genital tract
The usual dose is 3 g given every 4 hours (18 g/day) or 4 g given every 6 hours (16 g/day) depending on weight and the severity of the infection.

Dosage adjustment is required for patients with renal insufficiency (less than 30 mL/minute). For patients with a creatinine clearance of 10 to 30 mL/minute, administer 100% of the dose every 6 to 8 hours. For a creatinine clearance less than 10 mL/minute, administer 75% of the dose every 8 to 12 hours. In patients on hemodialysis, administer 3 g after dialysis, then 2 g every 12 hours. For patients with hepatic and renal failure, administer 2 g daily in one to two divided doses.

Monitor

Signs of infection (eg, temperature, white blood cell count with differential), culture and susceptibility, sodium, signs of bleeding, hypersensitivity reactions, and signs of central nervous system toxicity (neuromuscular hyperirritability and convulsions).

Ticarcillin is contraindicated for use in patients with a severe, documented allergy to penicillin antibiotics. It should be used cautiously in patients with allergies to cephalosporin or carbapenem antibiotics, as cross-reactivity may exist. Cross-reactivity with cephalosporins occurs in 3% to 15% of patients.

Protect from light: no

Special considerations

If concomitant aminoglycoside use is needed, administer at least 1 hour from the ticarcillin disodium and flush tubing prior to administration.

pH: 6.0 to 8.0

Stability

Reconstituted solution is clear, colorless, or pale yellow; stable at room temperature for at least 24 hours or for 72 hours with refrigeration.

Solution compatibility: D_5W and NS

Compatible drugs

Acyclovir sodium
Allopurinol sodium
Aztreonam
Cyclophosphamide
Diltiazem HCl
Famotidine
Filgrastim
Fludarabine phosphate
Heparin sodium
Hydromorphone HCl
IL-2

Insulin, regular
Magnesium sulfate
Melphalan HCl
Meperidine HCl
Morphine sulfate
Ondansetron HCl
Perphenazine
Sargramostim
Teniposide
Verapamil HCl
Vinorelbine tartrate

Incompatible drugs

Amrinone lactate
Chlorpromazine HCl
Dobutamine HCl
Erythromycin lactobionate
Fluconazole
Ganciclovir sodium
Gentamicin sulfate
Haloperidol lactate

Hydroxyzine HCl
Minocycline HCl
Papaverine HCl
Pentamidine isethionate
Pentazocine lactate
Promethazine HCl
Protamine sulfate
Quinidine gluconate

TICARCILLIN DISODIUM-CLAVULANATE POTASSIUM
Timentin®, SmithKline Beecham Pharmaceuticals

Method of administration
Intermittent intravenous infusion (over 30 minutes)

Dosage and administration
Standard: Ticarcillin disodium 3 g and clavulanic acid 0.1 g in 100 mL of D_5W

Ticarcillin disodium-clavulanate potassium is an extended-spectrum penicillin plus a β-lactamase inhibitor that is active against organisms susceptible to ticarcillin alone. In addition, because clavulanic acid can inhibit certain β-lactamases that generally inactivate ticarcillin, ticarcillin disodium-clavulanate potassium is active against many β-lactamase-producing organisms that are resistant to ticarcillin alone, including *Staphylococcus aureus, Bacteroides* sp, *Haemophilus influenzae, Escherichia coli,* and *Klebsiella pneumoniae.* Clavulanic acid generally acts as an irreversible, competitive inhibitor of β-lactamases. Synergism between the drugs does not occur against organisms that are susceptible to ticarcillin alone. Ticarcillin disodium-clavulanate potassium does have activity against *Pseudomonas aeruginosa*; however, it does not offer improved activity over piperacillin.

Treatment of septicemia and lower respiratory tract, urinary tract, skin and skin structure, and bone and joint infections
Administer 3.1 g (ticarcillin 3 g plus clavulanic acid 0.1 g) every 4 to 6 hours with a maximum of 24 g daily. For treatment of urinary tract infections, administer 3.1 g every 6 to 8 hours.

Dose or frequency adjustment is necessary in patients with renal insufficiency (creatinine clearance less than 30 mL/minute). In patients with a creatinine clearance of 10 to 30 mL/minute, administer at an interval of every 6 to 8 hours. With a creatinine clearance of less than 10 mL/minute, administer 75% of the dose every 8 to 12 hours. Patients receiving hemodialysis should receive an initial dose of ticarcillin disodium-clavulanate potassium of 3.1 g followed by a maintenance dose of 2 g every 12 hours. For patients with hepatic and renal failure, administer 2 g every 24 hours. Adjustment of dose is unnecessary in patients with hepatic impairment alone.

Monitor
Sign of infection (temperature, white blood cell count with differential), culture and susceptibility, hypersensitivity reactions, and signs of central nervous system toxicity (neuromuscular hyperirritability and convulsions).

Ticarcillin disodium-clavulanate potassium is contraindicated for use in patients with a documented allergy to penicillin antibiotics. It should be used cautiously in patients with allergies to cephalosporin or carbapenem antibiotics, as cross-reactivity may exist. Cross-reactivity with cephalosporins occurs in 3% to 15% of patients.

Protect from light: no

Special considerations
If concomitant aminoglycoside use is needed, administer at least 1 hour from ticarcillin disodium-clavulanate potassium and flush tubing prior to administration.

pH: 5.5 to 7.5

Stability
NS or D_5W is stable for 24 hours at room temperature and for 7 days in refrigeration.

Solution compatibility: D_5W, LR, and NS

Compatible drugs

Allopurinol sodium
Aztreonam
Cefepime HCl
Diltiazem HCl
Famotidine
Filgrastim
Fluconazole
Heparin sodium

Insulin, regular
Meperidine HCl
Morphine sulfate
Ondansetron HCl
Perphenazine
Sargramostim
Vinorelbine tartrate

Incompatible drugs

Amrinone lactate
Cefamandole nafate
Chlorpromazine HCl
Dobutamine HCl
Erythromycin lactobionate
Ganciclovir sodium

Haloperidol lactate
Hydroxyzine HCl
Pentazocine lactate
Promethazine HCl
Propofol
Protamine sulfate

TOBRAMYCIN SULFATE
Nebcin®, Eli Lilly and Company, and other manufacturers

Methods of administration
Intramuscular, intermittent intravenous infusion (over 30 minutes), intraventricular, or intrathecal

Dosing and administration
Standard: Dose/50 to 100 mL of D_5W or NS; larger (eg 500 mg) doses are diluted in 100 mL

Tobramycin is an aminoglycoside that is active against many aerobic gram-negative bacteria, including *Acinetobacter calcoaceticus, Escherichia coli, Haemophilus influenzae, Moraxella lacunata, Neisseria* sp, *Proteus* sp, *Serratia* sp, and *Pseudomonas* sp (including most strains of *Pseudomonas aeruginosa*). Tobramycin is usually less active than gentamicin against some gram-negative bacteria including *E coli* and *Serratia* sp. However, tobramycin is slightly more active against *P aeruginosa* than gentamicin. Tobramycin is active against some aerobic gram-positive bacteria, including *Staphylococcus aureus* and *Staphylococcus epidermidis*. Tobramycin is only minimally active against streptococci.

Treatment of suspected or documented gram-negative infections including bone, central nervous system, respiratory tract, and abdominal and urinary tract infections; endocarditis, septicemia; and skin and soft-tissue infections
Administer a loading dose of 2 mg/kg actual body weight (TBW) followed by a maintenance dose of 3 to 5 mg/kg in three equally divided doses every 8 to 12 hours. Typically administered for 7 to 10 days.

Dosage should be based on TBW and not ideal body weight (IBW). If patient is morbidly obese, then weight should be determined by using the formula IBW + 0.4 (TBW − IBW). A typical dose with adequate renal function (creatinine clearance less than 70 mL/minute) is 80 mg every 8 hours. Round dose to the nearest 10 mg. Pharmacokinetic monitoring is required to determine appropriate dose.

Once-a-day aminoglycoside regimens have also been used. A dose of 4 to 6 mg/kg is administered to patients who have an estimated creatinine clearance of at least 60 mL/minute. Subsequent doses are the same as the first. However, the interval is adjusted according to pharmacokinetic parameters to achieve a trough of less than 2 µg/mL.

Intrathecal and intraventricular administration: Doses of 3 to 10 mg are used for treatment of gram-negative bacillary meningitis. Tobramycin is typically administered in combination with systemic therapy.

Maintenance doses must be reduced in patients with renal insufficiency (95% of drug excreted unchanged by the kidneys). In patients with a creatinine clearance of 50 to 70 mL/minute, administer tobramycin every 12 hours. For a creatinine clearance of 30 to 50 mL/minute, administer every 18 hours. For a creatinine clearance of 15 to 30 mL/minute, give the drug daily. For a creatinine clearance less than 15 mL/minute, give an initial dose × 1, then dose when random level is less than 2 µg/mL. For patients receiving hemodialysis, dose after dialysis. Obtain serum drug levels as appropriate. No dosage adjustment recommended in patients with hepatic failure.

Monitor

Signs of infection (temperature, white blood cell count with differential), culture and susceptibility, signs of ototoxicity (auditory and vestibular [tinnitus, vertigo]), signs of nephrotoxicity (serum creatinine), and serum drug concentrations.

The risk of nephrotoxicity is dependent on several factors

Therapeutic drug monitoring considerations

Sample collection when patient at steady state:

Peak: 30 minutes after end of 30-minute infusion
60 minutes after intramuscular injection

Trough: within 30 minutes prior to dose

Therapeutic range:

Peak: 5 to 10 µg/mL

Trough: 0.5 to 2 µg/mL

---

and includes concomitant nephrotoxic drugs, prolonged elevated trough concentrations, age, hydration status, dose, and duration of treatment. Generally reversible upon discontinuation of drug.

Protect from light: no

Special considerations
If concomitant penicillin or cephalosporin use is needed, administer at least 1 hour from tobramycin and flush tubing prior to administration. Use preservative-free preparations for intrathecal and intraventricular administration.

pH: 3.0 to 6.5 (vial); 6 to 8 (constituted)

Stability
Stable at room temperature after reconstitution for at least 24 hours or for 96 hours with refrigeration; preservative-free solution should be used immediately.

Solution compatibility: D_5W, $D_{10}W$, NS, D_5NS, and LR

Compatible drugs

Acyclovir sodium	Hydromorphone HCl
Amiodarone HCl	IL-2
Amsacrine	Insulin, regular
Aztreonam	Labetalol HCl
Ciprofloxacin	Magnesium sulfate
Cyclophosphamide	Melphalan HCl
Diltiazem HCl	Meperidine HCl
Enalaprilat	Morphine sulfate
Esmolol HCl	Perphenazine
Filgrastim	Tacrolimus
Fluconazole	Teniposide
Fludarabine phosphate	Tolazoline HCl
Foscarnet sodium	Vinorelbine tartrate
Furosemide	Zidovudine

Incompatible drugs

Allopurinol sodium
Amphotericin B
Amrinone lactate
Azathioprine sodium
Cefamandole nafate
Cefazolin sodium
Cefepime HCl
Cefoperazone sodium
Cefotetan disodium
Ceftriaxone sodium
Chlorpromazine HCl
Clindamycin phosphate
Dexamethasone sodium
    phosphate
Folic acid
Ganciclovir sodium
Heparin sodium
Hetastarch
Mezlocillin sodium
Oxacillin sodium
Oxytocin
Pentamidine isethionate
Propofol
Pentobarbital sodium
Sargramostim

VANCOMYCIN HYDROCHLORIDE
Vancocin®, Eli Lilly and Company, and other manufacturers

Methods of administration
Intermittent intravenous infusion (over 60 to 90 minutes), intrathecal, intraventricular, and *not* intramuscular (risk of necrosis)

Dosing and administration
Standard: 500 mg/100 mL or 1000 mg/200 mL of D_5W or NS

Vancomycin is a glycopeptide antibiotic that is active against many gram-positive organisms, including staphylococci (including methicillin-resistant *Staphylococcus aureus*), *Streptococcus pyogenes, Streptococcus pneumoniae* (use for high level penicillin-resistant strains), enterococci, *Corynebacterium* sp, and *Clostridium* sp, including *Clostridium difficile.*

Treatment of skin and soft-tissue, bacterial endocarditis, bacteremia, pneumonia, bone and joint, graft, V-P shunt, and central nervous system infections
A typical dose for most patients with adequate renal function is 15 mg/kg given every 12 hours. Duration of therapy depends on type and severity of infection.

HICPAC Guidelines
The Hospital Infection Control Practices Advisory Committee (HICPAC) of the Centers for Disease Control and Prevention has developed guidelines to support appropriate use of vancomycin.
•Treatment of serious infections due to β-lactam-resistant gram-positive microorganisms
•Treatment of infections due to gram-positive microorganisms in patients with serious allergies to β-lactam antimicrobials
•When antibiotic-associated colitis (AAC) fails to respond to metronidazole or if AAC is severe and potentially life-threatening
•Prophylaxis, as recommended by the American Heart Association, for endocarditis following certain procedures in

patients at high risk for endocarditis

Prophylaxis for major surgical procedures involving implantation of prosthetic material or devices at institutions with a high rate of infections due to methicillin-resistant *Staphylococcus aureus* (MRSA) or methicillin-resistant *Staphylococcus epidermidis.*

Treatment of C difficile: 125 to 500 mg orally or through naso-gastric tube four times daily.

Intrathecal administration: Administer in doses up to 20 mg daily.

General

Dosage adjustment required for patients with renal insufficiency. In patients with a creatinine clearance of 30 to 65 mL/minute, increase the interval to every 24 hours. For patients with a creatinine clearance of 10 to 29 mL/minute, increase the interval to every 48 hours. If the creatinine clearance is less than 10 mL/minute, give initial dose $\times$ 1 and then dose when random level is 10 to 15 µg/mL. Typical dose is 1 g/week. Negligible amount of vancomycin is removed by hemodialysis unless using a high flux dialyzer. No changes required for patients with hepatic failure.

Monitor

Signs of infection (temperature, white blood cell count with differential), culture and susceptibility, serum creatinine (nephrotoxicity has occurred rarely and usually when given in combination with other nephrotoxic medications; early reports may have been due to an impurity in the formulation), ototoxicity (primarily associated with vancomycin levels greater than 80 µg/mL), hypersensitivity reactions, hypotension/flushing/pruritus of face, neck, and upper extremities (red man syndrome, which is often caused by infusing drug too rapidly), phlebitis (use large volume dilution), and serum drug concentrations.

Sample collection: (at steady state–3rd to 5th dose)

Peak:	60 minutes after end of 1-hour infusion
Trough:	within 30 minutes prior to dose

Therapeutic range*:

Peak:	30 to 40 µg/mL
Trough:	5 to 10 µg/mL

Troughs up to 15 µg/mL may be appropriate for central nervous system infections, osteomyelitis, and endocarditis.

* Vancomycin peaks are not routinely recommended.

Protect from light: no

Special considerations: none

pH: 2.5 to 4.5 (5% aqueous solution); 3 to 5 (in D_5W)

Stability: most stable at pH 3 to 5; stable at room temperature

Solution compatibility: D_5W, NS, D_5NS, $D_{10}W$, and LR

Compatible drugs

Acyclovir sodium	Magnesium sulfate
Allopurinol sodium	Melphalan HCl
Amiodarone HCl	Meperidine HCl
Amsacrine	Meropenem
Atracurium besylate	Morphine sulfate
Cyclophosphamide	Ondansetron HCl
Diltiazem HCl	Paclitaxel
Enalaprilat	Pancuronium bromide
Esmolol HCl	Perphenazine
Filgrastim	Sodium bicarbonate
Fluconazole	Tacrolimus
Fludarabine phosphate	Teniposide
Hydromorphone HCl	Vecuronium bromide
Insulin, regular	Vinorelbine tartrate
Labetalol HCl	Zidovudine

Incompatible drugs

Albumin
Aminophylline
Amphotericin B
Amrinone lactate
Azathioprine
Aztreonam
Cefazolin sodium
Cefepime HCl
Cefoperazone sodium
Cefotaxime sodium
Cefoxitin
Ceftazidime
Chloramphenicol sodium
    succinate
Dexamethasone sodium
    phosphate
Epoetin alfa
Foscarnet sodium
Furosemide
Ganciclovir sodium
Heparin sodium
Idarubicin HCl
Ketorolac tromethamine
Methicillin sodium
Mezlocillin
Phenobarbital sodium
Phenytoin sodium
Piperacillin sodium-
    tazobactam sodium
Propofol
Sargramostim
Secobarbital sodium
Streptokinase
Urokinase
Warfarin sodium

VECURONIUM BROMIDE
Norcuron®, Organon Inc., and other manufacturers

Methods of administration
Direct intravenous injection (undiluted), intermittent intravenous infusion, and *not* intramuscular

Dosing and administration
Standard: 100 mg/250 mL of D_5W or NS (concentrated solutions of 100 mg/100 mL)

Immobilization for mechanical ventilation
Vecuronium is an intermediate-acting, nondepolarizing, neuromuscular blocker (onset of effect: 3 to 5 minutes; duration: 35 to 45 minutes, depending on dose). Patients can receive a loading dose of 0.075 to 0.1 mg/kg (5 to 10 mg) by direct intravenous injection over 15 to 30 seconds. Blockade can be maintained at a dose of 1 µg/kg/minute as an initial continuous infusion. Titrate by increments of 0.25 µg/kg/minute at 1-hour intervals based on peripheral nerve stimulation.

Pancuronium is the preferred neuromuscular blocker for most critically ill patients. Vecuronium is preferred for those patients with cardiac disease or hemodynamic instability in whom tachycardia may be deleterious. (See practice parameters for sustained neuromuscular blockade in the suggested readings.)

DO NOT PARALYZE PATIENT WITHOUT ADEQUATE SEDATION. Need to coadminister with medications that provide sedation, analgesia, or amnesia. Use precaution with pressure points on the eyes or skin, and provide prophylaxis for thrombosis. Indications for neuromuscular blocking agents in the intensive care unit include endotracheal intubation, status epilepticus, status asthmaticus, adult respiratory distress syndrome, neuromuscular toxins, tetanus, and hypothermia.

Dosage adjustments
Renal: No dosage or interval generally required for short-term use in patients with renal insufficiency. Some accumulation of

the active metabolite (3-desacetyl-vecuronium) may occur with prolonged use, and the maintenance dose should be reduced accordingly (based on response to train-of-four monitoring).

Hepatic: Dosage adjustment necessary (decrease maintenance infusion rate) in patients with hepatic insufficiency.

Monitor

Neuromuscular blockade (peripheral nerve stimulation with train-of-four monitoring every 4 to 8 hours with a goal of 2 to 4 twitches), blood pressure (hypotension), heart rate (tachycardia or bradycardia), manifestations of histamine release (eg, skin flushing, erythema, and pruritus), and convulsions (rare and usually in patients with predisposing factors such as head trauma).

Several risk factors place a patient at increased risk of prolongation of neuromuscular blockade: accumulation of drug or metabolite, electrolyte imbalance (hypokalemia, hypomagnesemia, and hypocalcemia), and medications including calcium channel blockers, corticosteroids, anti-arrhythmics (eg, procainamide and quinidine), antibiotics (eg, aminoglycosides), and immunosuppressants. Chronic use of phenytoin or carbamazepine may result in resistance to neuromuscular blockade.

Generally no histamine-release hypotension or vagal-block tachycardia. Generally considered to be a safe alternative in patients who are cardiovascularly compromised.

Protect from light: no

Special considerations: none

pH: 4

Stability

Do not mix with medications that have a basic pH; stable for 24 hours at room temperature in all compatible diluents.

Solution compatibility: D$_5$W, NS, D$_5$NS, and LR

Compatible drugs

Aminophylline
Cefazolin sodium
Cefuroxime sodium
Cimetidine HCl
Dobutamine HCl
Dopamine HCl
Epinephrine HCl
Esmolol HCl
Fentanyl citrate
Fluconazole
Gentamicin sulfate
Heparin sodium
Hydrocortisone sodium
  succinate
Isoproterenol HCl
Lorazepam
Midazolam HCl
Morphine sulfate
Nitroglycerin
Nitroprusside sodium
Ranitidine HCl
Trimethoprim-
  sulfamethoxazole
Vancomycin HCl

Incompatible drugs

Diazepam
Etomidate
Propofol

VERAPAMIL HYDROCHLORIDE
Isoptin®, Knoll Laboratories, and other manufacturers

Methods of administration
Direct intravenous injection (over 2 to 3 minutes), and continuous intravenous infusion

Dosing and administration
Standard: 100 mg/250 mL of D_5W or NS (maximum: 100 mg/100 mL)

Supraventricular tachycardia and to slow ventricular rate in atrial fibrillation or flutter
Administer 2.5 to 5 mg by direct intravenous injection over 2 to 3 minutes. Repeat if necessary with 5 to 10 mg within 15 to 30 minutes after initial intravenous injection. Alternatively, 5 mg may be given every 15 minutes (maximum total dose of 30 mg). Administer a continuous infusion of 5 mg/hour (1.2 µg/kg/minute) and titrate to control ventricular rate below 100 beats/minute by increments of 0.5 to 1 µg/kg minute at 6-hour intervals (maximum approximately 5 µg/kg/minute). Patients with an ejection fraction of 30% to 50%, or those with mild hepatic disease may require 0.5 to 1.0 µg/kg/minute). Avoid in patients with severe left ventricular dysfunction (ejection fraction less than 30%) because of negative inotropic effects.

Reduce dose 20% to 50% in patients with cirrhosis. In patients with a creatinine clearance of less than 10 mL/minute, administer 50% to 75% of normal dose. Since the drug is not dialyzable (hemodialysis or peritoneal dialysis), supplemental dose unnecessary.

Monitor
Heart rate (bradycardia, which is most frequently seen in patients with conduction abnormalities), ECG (AV nodal block), blood pressure (hypotension, which is seen most frequently during or after direct intravenous injection), headache, dizziness, and constipation.

Inhibits nonrenal clearance of digoxin, leading to a significant rise in digoxin serum concentrations.

Pretreatment with calcium gluconate (1 g intravenously) may reduce the incidence and severity of hypotension without affecting the effectiveness of the drug.

Protect from light: yes

Special considerations: none

pH: 4.1 to 6

Stability: stable at pH range of 3 to 6 (precipitate forms at pH >6)

Solution compatibility: D_5W, NS, D_5NS, LR, and ½NS

Compatible drugs

Amrinone lactate	Meperidine HCl
Ciprofloxacin	Methicillin sodium
Dobutamine HCl	Milrinone
Dopamine HCl	Penicillin G potassium
Famotidine	Piperacillin sodium
Hydralazine HCl	Ticarcillin disodium

Incompatible drugs

Albumin	Ganciclovir
Aminophylline	Metronidazole HCl
Amphotericin B	Mezlocillin sodium
Ampicillin sodium	Nafcillin sodium
Ampicillin sodium-sulbactam sodium	Oxacillin sodium
Azathioprine sodium	Pentobarbital sodium
Cefoperazone sodium	Phenobarbital sodium
Ceftazidime (sodium bicarbonate)	Propofol
Folic acid	Sodium bicarbonate
Furosemide	Trimethoprim-sulfamethoxazole

SUGGESTED READINGS

Abramowicz M, ed. Antimicrobial prophylaxis in surgery. *Med Lett Drugs Ther*. 1992;34:5-8.

Adams HP, Brott TG, Furlan AJ, et al. Guidelines for thrombolytic therapy for acute stroke: a supplement to the guidelines for the management of patients with acute ischemic stroke. *Circulation*. 1996;94:1167-1174.

Bodey GP. Azole antifungal agents. *Clin Infect Dis*. 1992;14(suppl 1):S161-S169.

Califf RM, White HD, Van de Werf F, et al. One-year results from the Global Utilization of Streptokinase and TPA for Occluded Coronary Arteries (GUSTO-I) trial. *Circulation*. 1996;94:1233-1238.

Condon RE, Wittmann DH. The use of antibiotics in general surgery. *Curr Probl Surg*. 1991;28(12):807-907.

Drugs for cardiac arrhythmias. *Med Lett Drugs Ther*. 1996;38:75-82.

Guest TM, Ramanathan AV, Tuteur PG, Schechtman KB, Ladenson JH, Jaffe AS. Myocardial injury in critically ill patients, a frequently unrecognized complication. *JAMA*. 1995;273:1945-1949.

Guidelines for the management of patients with acute ischemic stroke. A statement for healthcare professionals from a special writing group of the Stroke Council, American Heart Association. *Stroke*. 1994;25(9):1901-1914.

Hacke W, Kaste M, Fieschi C, et al. Intravenous thrombolysis with recombinant tissue plasminogen activator for acute hemispheric stroke, The European Cooperative Acute Stroke Study. *JAMA*. 1995;274:1017-1025.

Indications for fibrinolytic therapy in suspected acute myocardial infarction: collaborative overview of early mortality and major morbidity results from all randomised trials of more than 1000 patients. Fibrinolytic Therapy Trialists' (FTT) Collaborative Group. *Lancet.* 1994;343:311-322.

Jordan KG. Status epilepticus. A perspective from the neuroscience intensive care unit. *Neurosurgery Clin N Am.* 1994;5:671-686.

Lewis RT, Weigand FM, Mamazza J, Lloyd-Smith W, Tataryn D. Should antibiotic prophylaxis be used routinely in clean surgical procedures: a tentative yes. *Surgery.* 1995;118:742-747.

Leroy O, Santre C, Beuscart C, et al. A five-year study of severe community-acquired pneumonia with emphasis on prognosis in patients admitted to an intensive care unit. *Intensive Care Med.* 1995;21:24-31.

Lipsky MS. Management of diabetic ketoacidosis. *Am Fam Physician.* 1994;49:1607-1612.

Nguyen MH, Peacock JE Jr, Tanner DC, et al. Therapeutic approaches in patients with candidemia. *Arch Intern Med.* 1995;155:2429-2435.

Nichols RL. Surgical wound infection. *Am J Med.* 1991;91(3B):54S-64S.

Rainey TG, Read CA. Pharmacology of colloids and crystalloids. In, Chernow B, ed. *The Pharmacologic Approach to the Critically Ill Patient.* Baltimore, Md: Williams and Wilkins; 1996; chap 15, section 2: 272-287.

Rex JH, Bennett JE, Sugar AM, et al. A randomized trial comparing fluconazole with amphotericin B for the treatment of candidemia in patients without neutropenia. Candidemia Study Group and the National Institute. *N Engl J Med.* 1994;331:1325-1330.

Rumbak MJ, Kitabchi AE. Diabetic ketoacidosis: etiology, pathology and treatment. *Compr Ther*. 1991:17(7); 46-49.

Savino JA, Agarwal N, Wry P, Policastro A, Cerabona T, Austria L. Routine prophylactic antifungal agents (clotrimazole, keto-conazole, and nystatin) in nontransplant/nonburned critically ill surgical and trauma patients. *J Trauma*. 1994;36(1):20-26.

Sherman DG, Dyken ML Jr, Gent M, Harrison JG, Hart RG, Mohr JP. Antithrombotic therapy for cerebrovascular disorders. An update. *Chest*. 1995;108(4):444S-456S.

The choice of antibacterial drugs. *Med Lett Drugs Ther*. 1996;38:25-34.

The problem of sepsis, an expert report of the European Society of Intensive Care Medicine. Intensive Care Medicine. 1994; 20: 300-304.

The Task Force on the Management of Acute Myocardial Infarction of the European Society of Cardiology. Acute myocardial infarction: pre-hospital and in-hospital management. *Eur Heart J*. 1996;17:43-63.

Treatment of convulsive status epilepticus. Recommendations of the Epilepsy Foundation of America's Working Group on Status Epilepticus. *JAMA*. 1993; 270: 854-859.

Wunderink RG. Pneumonia in the intensive care unit. *Clin Chest Med*. 1995;016(1):1-223.

DRUG COMPATIBILITY TABLE

This table has been developed as an easy-to-use resource to find the information on compatibility on 46 medications commonly used in the intensive care unit.

- Medications are considered to be compatible (C) if the following exists:

    Data are available that support COMPATIBILITY when the two medications are administered concomitantly through a Y-site.
- Medications are considered to be incompatible (I) if the following exists:

    Data are available that these two medications are physically or chemically INCOMPATIBLE when tested for additive, syringe, or Y-site compatibility.

These data are meant to be used for general purposes, the reader is referred to the original data when applicable.

C	= Compatible
I	= Incompatible
Blank box	= No information available
X	= Same drug

	1	2	3	4	5	6	7	8	9	10	11	12	13	14
1. Aminophyline	X	I	C		C				I	I	I		C	I
2. Amiodarone	I	X		C							C	C		
3. Amrinone	C		X	C	C	I		C		I	C	C		C
4. Bretylium		C	C	X					C		C			
5. Cimetidine	C		C		X				C				C	
6. Dexamethasone			I			X	I			I	I			
7. Diazepam						I	X				C			I
8. Digoxin			C					X	C		I			
9. Diltiazem	I			C	C		I	C	X		C	C		C
10. Diphenhydramine	I		I		I					X				
11. Dobutamine	I	C	C	C		I	C	I	C		X	C	C	
12. Dopamine		C	C						C		C	X	C	
13. Enalaprilat	C				C						C	C	X	
14. Epinephrine	I		C				I		C					X
15. Erythromycin		C				I			C				C	
16. Esmolol	C		I		C	I	I		C			C	C	
17. Famotidine	C		C	C		C		C			C	C	C	C
18. Fentanyl													C	
19. Furosemide			I		I		I		I	I	I			
20. Haloperidol	I			I	C	I				I	C	C		
21. Heparin		I	I		C	C	I	C	I	C	I	C	C	C
22. Hydromorphone						I	I							
23. Insulin, human	I	C	I					C	I	I	C	I		
24. Isoproterenol	I	C	C	C										
25. Labetalol	C	C			C	I					C	C	C	
26. Lidocaine		C	C						C		C	C	C	I
27. Lorazepam									C					
28. Mannitol			I											
29. Methylprednisolone			C						I	I			C	
30. Metaclopramide			I						C					
31. Metoprolol														
32. Midazolam	I	C				I						C		
33. Morphine	C	C	I			C		C	C			C	C	
34. Nitroglycerin		C	C						C		C	C		
35. Nitroprusside			C						C	I	C	C	C	
36. Norepinephrine	I	C	C						C			C		
37. Pancuronium	C				C		I				C	C		C
38. Pentobarbital			I		I						I	I		I
39. Phenobarbital			I		I						I	I	C	I
40. Phenylephrine		C	C											
41. Procainamide		C	C	I					C					
42. Propofol	I		I	I	I	I	I	I		I	I	I		I
43. Ranitidine	C			C			I		C		C	C	C	
44. Sodium bicarbonate		I	I			C			I	I	I	I		I
45. Vecuronium	C				C		I				C	C		C
46. Verapamil	I		C								C	C		

	15	16	17	18	19	20	21	22	23	24	25	26	27	28
1. Aminophyline		C	C			I			I	I	C			
2. Amiodarone	C	C					I		C	C	C	C		
3. Amrinone		I	C		I		I		I	C		C		I
4. Bretylium			C			I				C				
5. Cimetidine		C				I	C	C			C			
6. Dexamethasone	I	I	C			I	C	I			I			
7. Diazepam		I			I		I	I						
8. Digoxin			C				C		C					
9. Diltiazem	C	C			I		I		I			C	C	
10. Diphenhydramine					I	I	C		I					
11. Dobutamine			C		I	C	I		C		C	C		
12. Dopamine		C	C			C	C		I		C	C		
13. Enalaprilat	C	C	C	C			C				C	C		
14. Epinephrine			C				C					I		
15. Erythromycin	X	C	C		I		C	C			C			
16. Esmolol	C	X	C	C	I		C		C		C			
17. Famotidine	C	C	X		C	C	C		C	C	C	C		
18. Fentanyl		C		X			C				C			
19. Furosemide	I	I	C		X	I	C			I	I			
20. Haloperidol			C		I	X	I					C	C	
21. Heparin	C	C	C	C	C	I	X		C	C	C	C		
22. Hydromorphone	C							X						
23. Insulin, human		C	C				C		X	I	I			
24. Isoproterenol			C		I		C		I	X				
25. Labetalol	C	C	C	C	I		C		I		X	C		
26. Lidocaine			C			C	C				C	X		
27. Lorazepam							C						X	
28. Mannitol														X
29. Methylprednisolone		I	C			I	C		C					
30. Metoclopramide	I		C		I		C							
31. Metoprolol	I													
32. Midazolam		C	C	C	I				C		C			
33. Morphine	C	C	C		I		C		C		C	C		
34. Nitroglycerin		C	C			C	C		C		C	C		
35. Nitroprusside	I	C	C			I	C		C		C	C		
36. Norepinephrine			C		I	C	C		I		C	I		
37. Pancuronium		C		C			C			C			C	
38. Pentobarbital	I	I		I		I		I	C	I		I		
39. Phenobarbital	I	I				I		I		I		I		
40. Phenylephrine			C			C			I					
41. Procainadmide		I	I				C							
42. Propofol		I	I				I			I	I	I	I	
43. Ranitidine		C					C				C			
44. Sodium bicarbonate			C			I	C	I	C	I	I			
45. Vecuronium		C		C			C			C			C	
46. Verapamil			C		I									

	29	30	31	32	33	34	35	36	37	38	39	40	41	42	43	44	45	46
1.				I	C			I	C					I	C		C	I
2.					C	C	C		C				C	C		I		
3.	C	I			I	C	C	C		I	I	C	C	I		I		C
4.														I	I	C		
5.								C	I	I				I			C	
6.				I	C									I		C		
7.									I					I	I	I	I	
8.					C									I				
9.	I	C			C	C	C	C					C		C			
10.	I						I			I	I			I		I		
11.						C	C		C	I	I			I	C	I	C	C
12.				C	C	C	C	C	C					I	C	I	C	C
13.	C				C		C				C				C			
14.									C	I	I			I		I	C	
15.		I	I		C		I			I	I							
16.	I			C	C	C	C	C	C	I	I		I	I	C		C	
17.	C	C		C	C	C	C	C				C	C	I		C		C
18.				C					C	I							C	
19.		I		I	I			I										I
20.	I					C	I	C		I	I	C				I		
21.	C	C		C	C	C	C	C					C	I	C	C	C	
22.										I	I					I		
23.	C			C	C	C	C	I		C		I				C		
24.									C	I	I					I	C	
25.				C	C	C	C	C						I	C	I		
26.					C	C	C	I		I	I			I				
27.								C						I			C	
28.																		
29.	X			C										I		C		
30.		X		C										I		I		
31.			X	C														
32.				X	C	C	C	C	C	I	I			I	I	I	C	
33.	C	C	C	C	X	C	C	C	C	I	I			I	C	C	C	
34.				C	C	X	C		C					I	C		C	
35.				C	C	C	X		C					I			C	
36.				C	C			X		I	I					I	I	
37.				C	C	C	C		X	I	I			I	C			
38.				I	I			I	I	X				I	I	I		I
39.				I	I			I	I		X			I	I			I
40.												X		I				
41.													X		C			
42.	I	I		I	I	I	I	I		I	I	I	I	X	I	I	I	I
43.				I	C	C			C	I	I		C	I	X		C	
44.	C	I		I	C			I		I				I		X		I
45.				C	C	C	C							I	C	I	X	
46.										I	I			I		I		X

SUGGESTED READINGS FOR TABLE

Bosso JA, Rince RA, Fox JL. Compatibility of ondansetron hydrochloride with fluconazole, ceftazidime, aztreonam, and cefazolin sodium under simulated Y-site conditions. *Am J Hosp Pharm*. 1994;51(3):389-391.

Catania PN, ed. *King Guide to Parenteral Mixtures*. St. Louis, Mo: Pacemarq, Inc.; 1995.

Choi JS, Burm JP, Jhee SS, Chin A, Ulrich RW, Gill MA. Stability of piperacillin sodium-tazobactam sodium and ranitidine hydrochloride in 0.9% sodium chloride injection during simulated Y-site administration. *Am J Hosp Pharm*. 1994;51:2273-2276.

Colucci RD, Cobuzzi LE, Halpern NA. Visual compatibility of esmolol hydrochloride and various injectable drugs during simulated Y-site injection. *Am J Hosp Pharm*. 1988;45:630-632.

Colucci RD, Cobuzzi LE, Halpern NA. Visual compatibility of labetalol hydrochloride injection with various injectable drugs during simulated Y-site injection. *Am J Hosp Pharm*. 1988;45:135-138.

Elmore RL, Contois ME, Kelly J, Noe A, Poirier A. Stability and compatibility of admixtures of intravenous ciprofloxacin and selected drugs. *Clin Ther*. 1996;18(2):246-255.

Farquhar Zanetti LA. Visual compatibility of diltiazem with commonly used injectable drugs during simulated Y-site administration. *Am J Hosp Pharm*. 1992;49:1911-1912.

Fong PA, Ward J. Visual compatibility of intravenous famotidine with selected drugs. *Am J Hosp Pharm*. 1989;46:125-126.

Hassan E, Leslie J, Martir-Herrero ML. Stability of labetalol hydrochloride with selected critical care drugs during simulated Y-site injection. *Am J Hosp Pharm.* 1994;51:2143 -2145.

Hutchings SR, Rusho WJ, Tyler LS. Compatibility of cefmetazole sodium with commonly used drugs during Y-site delivery. *Am J Health Syst Pharm.* 1996;53(18):2185-2188.

Inagaki K, Takagi J, Lor E, Lee KJ, Nii L, Gill MA. Stability of fluconazole in commonly used intravenous antibiotic solutions. *Am J Hosp Pharm.* 1993;50:1206-1208.

Jay GT, Fanikos J, Souney PF. Visual compatibility of famotidine with commonly used critical-care medications during simulated Y-site injection. *Am J Hosp Pharm.* 1988;45:1556-1557.

Lor E, Sheybani T, Takagi J. Visual compatibility of fluconazole with commonly used injectable drugs during simulated Y-site administration. *Am J Hosp Pharm.* 1991;48:744-746.

Mantong ML, Marquardt ED. Visual compatibility of midazolam hydrochloride with selected drugs during simulated Y-site injection. *Am J Health Syst Pharm.* 1995;52(22):2567-2568.

Marquardt ED, Lam SSY. Visual compatibility of fentanyl citrate with selected drugs during simulated Y-site injection. *Am J Hosp Pharm.* 1994;51:811-812.

Mayron D, Gennaro AR. Stability and compatibility of granisetron hydrochloride in iv solutions and oral liquids and during simulated Y-site injection with selected drugs. *Am J Health Syst Pharm.* 1996;53(3):294-304.

Patel PR. Compatibility of meropenem with commonly used injectable drugs. *Am J Health Syst Pharm.* 1996;53(23):2853-2855.

Pugh CB, Pabis DJ, Rodriguez C. Visual compatibility of morphine sulfate and meperidine hydrochloride with other injectable drugs during simulated Y-site injection. *Am J Hosp Pharm.* 1991;48:123-125.

Savitsky ME. Visual compatibility of neuromuscular blocking agents with various injectable drugs during simulated Y-site injection. *Am J Hosp Pharm.* 1990;47:820-821.

Trissel LA. *Handbook on Injectable Drugs.* Bethesda, Md: American Society of Health-Systems Pharmacists, Inc.; 1996.

Trissel LA, Leissing NC. *Trissel's Tables.* Lake Forest, Ill: MultiMatrix, Inc.; 1996.

Trissel LA, Martinez P. Compatibility of piperacillin sodium plus tazobactam with selected drugs during simulated Y-site injection. *Am J Hosp Pharm.* 1994;51:672-678.

Tucker DR, Sieradzan R. Visual compatibility of ciprofloxacin lactate with five broad-spectrum antimicrobial agents during simulated Y-site injection. *Am J Hosp Pharm.* 1988;45:1910-1911.

Yamashita SK, Walker SE, Choudhury T, Iazzetta J. Compatibility of selected critical care drugs during simulated Y-site administration. *Am J Health Syst Pharm.* 1996;53(9):1048-1051.

GENERIC/BRAND NAME INDEX

313

THERAPEUTIC CATEGORY INDEX

315

Miscellaneous

* **Listed in more than one category**

THE INJECTABLE DRUG REFERENCE

Use this form to order additional copies

☐ Please enter the number of copies you wish to order clearly

Prices	Per Copy
Regular price	$ 29.95
Shipping & handling	1.25
	$ 31.20

Total number of copies × $31.20 _____

NJ residents add 6% sales tax _____

($1.80 per book)

Total cost of order $_____

☐ Enclosed is my check or money order payable to Bioscientific Resources, Inc.

☐ Please issue an invoice with shipping & handling included. Enclosed is our purchase order, number: _____

Please ship the book(s) to the following address: *(print clearly)*

❑ Home Address   or   ❑ Business Address

Name _____Title _____

Institution/Department _____

Address _____

City _____State _____Zip Code _____

Telephone _____

Please mail this form to: **Bioscientific Resources, Inc.**
P.O. Box 8735
Woodcliff Lake, NJ 07675-8735

Or, fax form and purchase order to (201) 573-1054